How to Raise a Mindful Eater

Other books by Maryann Jacobsen:

The Family Dinner Solution

From Picky to Powerful

Fearless Feeding

What Does Your Tummy Say?

Praise for *How to Raise a Mindful Eater*

"Finally! Maryann's *How to Raise a Mindful Eater* takes feeding kids to the next level — intentional and thoughtful approaches to raise kids who eat with thought and intention."
— Jill Castle, MS, RDN, pediatric nutrition expert and author of *Eat Like a Champion*

"Maryann Jacobsen has written an extremely helpful book in which she explains the truth about nutrition, and gives guidelines on how to raise kids to have a healthy attitude towards food, facilitating intuitive eating and mindfulness."
— Dr. Nina Savelle-Rocklin, psychoanalyst, author, eating disorder specialist

"What I love about Maryann's advice on feeding kids is that she combines in-depth research along with her own experience as a mother to provide a compassionate and sensible but evidence-based approach."
— Sally Kuzemchak, MS, RD, creator of RealMomNutrition.com

"Maryann Jacobsen MS, RD has balanced science, research and common sense to write a book about mindful eating that will completely transform your families diet. This book is a fabulous way to bring mindful eating fully into the home."
— Megrette Fletcher M.Ed., RD, CDE, co-founder of The Center for Mindful Eating and author of *Discover Mindful Eating for Kids*

"Maryann Jacobsen's latest book *How to Raise a Mindful Eater* guides you toward developing a way of looking at feeding your children which is not reactionary. Instead, she shows you how to take the big picture into consideration, for the present moment and the future. A must-read for all parents, whether your children are little or big!"
— Katja Leccisi, MS, RDN, author of *How to Feed Your Kids* and *Questions and Answers About Your Baby's First Foods*

"*How to Raise a Mindful Eater* offers sound, sane and compassionate advice for shepherding kids to a healthy relationship with food and their bodies, and at the same time reminds the adults how we can benefit from the mindful practices of self-care and self-love that Maryann has so beautifully laid out for us all. This book is truly a must-read!"
— Tricia Nelson, Certified Coach and author of *Heal Your Hunger*

"If you've ever wondered about the best ways to feed your child - and what parent hasn't - you'll find answers here. Maryann Jacobsen's insightful and practical book will guide you in helping your children develop a healthy relationship with food and their bodies."
— Judith Matz, LCSW, author of *Amanda's Big Dream* and co-author of *The Diet Survivor's Handbook*

"*How to Raise A Mindful Eater* is such a wonderful resource for parents looking to give their kids a healthy relationship with food from the get-go. Maryann gives a great discussion of the studies that support the book's recommendations, and she writes in a really approachable way." — Kara Buetel, MS, Nutrition Coach and creator of RaisingNutrition.com

How to Raise a Mindful Eater

8 Powerful Principles for Transforming Your Child's Relationship with Food

Maryann Jacobsen, MS, RD

Printed in the United States of America

First Edition

ISBN-13: 978-1541129283
ISBN-10: 1541129288

www.MaryannJacobsen.com/RMIBooks

DEDICATION

This book is dedicated to my husband, Dan. Without your support and love, there would be no books. I love you!

CONTENTS

ACKNOWLEDGMENTS

I want to thank all the people who helped make this book a reality. First, my blog readers who read through the manuscript and offered feedback. I always am amazed how much better you make my books. Next are the parents who took the time to share their amazing stories, especially Marci. You have helped more families than you will ever know. And a special thank you to all the experts who offered their advice. I only hope to shine more light on your work that has already made the world a healthier place. Thanks to Rob Bignell and Arnetta Jackson, for attention to detail in editing. And what would I do without my family who puts up with all that goes on when I'm writing a book? Your support and love is what keeps me going.

INTRODUCING A NEW WAY TO SEE FOOD

"No problem can be solved from the same level of consciousness that created it."
-Albert Einstein

Marci's first child was born healthy, just over seven pounds. Things quickly changed as her daughter's appetite and weight grew faster than the doctors wanted. Marci was given advice early on to limit formula feeding, so she did. When her daughter turned two, she noticed something wasn't quite right. She was never happy when she was done eating. But staying with the tried-and-true advice, Marci kept her daughter to child-size portions. When mom wasn't around to control her daughter's eating, she ate large amounts. Outsiders began to comment on how much she ate, sharing with Marci that "She had four string cheeses" during snack time. Marci began to feel self-conscious and even found her daughter sneaking into food drawers.

Marci found herself in a no-win situation. Being the 'food police' took a lot of work, with no end in sight. Like a lot of parents in her shoes, she didn't know there was a very different way of approaching her daughter's eating. This book is about this "other way" that, unfortunately, few families know about. It's an approach to eating – and feeding – that actually solves eating-related challenges, and enables your family to create a healthy relationship with food.

The Second Arrow

The Buddha once asked a student, "If a person is struck by an arrow, is it painful?" The student replied, "It is." The Buddha then asked, "If the person is struck by a second arrow, is that even more painful?" The student replied again, "It is." The Buddha then explained, "In life, we cannot always control the first arrow. However, the second arrow is our reaction to the first. The second arrow is optional."

To explain suffering, this parable uses the example of two arrows. There's the first arrow that causes pain. But it's really the second arrow that is responsible for suffering. We tend to forget that the second arrow, our reaction to what happens, is something very much in our control. When it comes to food and health, the first arrow has been clearly defined to us in a fearful way. The Standard American Diet is killing us. People eat too much sugar, fat, and salt, and not enough fruits, vegetables, and whole grains. Rising obesity is contributing to chronic disease and parents may even outlive their kids. Food companies not only spend time making food addicting, they advertise it constantly. We've gotten the message loud and clear: *Things look grim.*

The second arrow, the reaction, has also been fear-based in the form of a food fight. If food caused the first arrow, forcing food to change must be the answer. New diets come faster than cars do on a freeway, each one promising to be our health and weight savior. Government officials have joined in this food fight too, attempting to tax bad food, requiring calorie counts on menus, and banning nutrition-poor food and drinks in school.

Food has been examined, feared, loved, controlled, abused, and has sadly become a point of contention for many people. The simple pleasure of eating now has so much baggage and causes so much suffering. There's plenty of evidence that we are just spinning our wheels with this fix-the-food strategy. A 2015 article in The New York Times, "Obesity Rises Despite All Efforts to Fight It, US Officials Say," includes interviews with experts dumbfounded that obesity has gone up despite decreases in soda, sugar, and calories.[1] And what about those diets? While short-term weight loss results, over time studies show diets actually predict future weight gain.[2]

The reason none of these strategies work is because food is not the answer. What and how much we eat is really just a symptom of something else entirely. It's the second arrow, because we are treating symptoms instead of causes.

Marci fell into the second-arrow trap restricting her child's food intake only to add more layers of pain and suffering. She decided to take a different approach after reading books and getting professional help. Slowly but surely she changed how she reacted to her child. Instead of fear, she began trusting her daughter around food and learned new strategies. "It was scary at first because she ate like crazy but then there was a moment my daughter pushed her plate away with food on it," she said. "I started to see it was working and noticed my daughter stopped thinking of food between eating time."

The secret to Marci's success is that she dealt with the key factor that ultimately determines what and how much people eat: *their relationship with food.* After going through a similar process as the one outlined in this book, she now feels good about her daughter's eating. And she was able to kick her role as food police to the curb.

The Incomplete Food Story

A major part of the problem with the familiar story of food and weight gone bad is it's incomplete. Yes, the industrial revolution brought significant changes to the food supply, but it was the shift in people's relationship with food around the 1970s that did the most damage. This is when cooking and family meals took a backseat and a record number of women joined the workforce. Food companies and restaurants took over this important job, and making food at home dropped in favor of convenience. Frozen dinners and other convenience foods popped up everywhere and eating out almost doubled from 18 percent in the late 1970s to 32 percent in 2005-2008.[3] Eating on the go increased, with snacking gradually replacing sit-down meals.[4] The creation of those convenient TV stands allowed families to eat and watch their favorite show. It's no wonder the sharpest increase in obesity occurred to those born after 1971.[5]

Experts like to go on about how food has changed, but what preceded and contributed to this change was a new way of relating to food. For the first time in human history, food dropped as a priority and people began to eat on autopilot. In other words, the era of mindless eating was born.

At the time, no one could foresee the unintended consequences of this paradigm shift. I don't think anyone felt guilty for popping in frozen meals or allowing TV stands at dinnertime (I know my mom didn't!). In fact, this was a liberating time, as it freed women from the burden of preparing food. This liberation didn't last long, as the obesity crisis emerged, first in whispers but eventually to the loud roar we hear today. In 2001, the Surgeon General's "Call to Action to Prevent and Decrease Overweight and Obesity" made obesity a public health priority after statistics showed that more than half of adults were obese or overweight.[6] In 2010, First Lady Michelle Obama spearheaded Let's Move, an initiative with the ambitious goal of ending childhood obesity "in a generation."[7]

The free market, including the media, food companies, books, and commercial weight-loss programs, have been quick to come up with their own solutions to people's weight woes. The media discovered that sensationalized articles about obesity and "bad-for-you" foods draws readers. In fact, obesity-related news stories shot up from 500 to 6,500 from 1991 to 2005![8] In 1994, the FDA regulated claims on food packages providing a framework to call food "healthy," "low fat," and "sugar-free." Less-than-nutritious products appeared in grocery stores along with each diet trend, like fat-free Snack Wells in the 1980s and gluten-free baked goods in 2010. Diet books and commercial weight-loss programs have exploded in popularity because they help people lose weight quickly, even though keeping the weight off remains a challenge.

Despite all this effort, the consumption of nutritious foods like fruits and vegetables and levels of physical activity remain far below recommendations. In short, there has been no real long-term change to people's health-related behavior. It's not because people are lazy, lack willpower, or tasty food is too tempting. It's that we never healed our relationship with food, the real instigator behind the way people eat. I should know because I've been there.

From Mindless to Mindful

I am a registered dietitian but my education is not what taught me how to eat in a balanced way. Although learning about nutrition was helpful, I remained clueless about eating in moderation. If ice cream was in the house, I HAD to finish it. If I gave in and had one cookie, I'd end up having more than I could count.

Like everyone's food relationship, mine began developing as a child. My dad grew up poor and ate any and all leftovers because he hated to see food go to waste. My mom, who also struggled with eating, tried to keep the kitchen stocked, but with five children running around, my siblings and I fought over every last cookie and donut crumb. In high school, I lost weight by cutting how much I ate in half, so I could be thin and accepted. When I got to college, I thought majoring in nutrition would give me answers, but when I still couldn't eat certain foods in moderation, I just assumed it was hard for everyone. In the back of my mind, I thought if I kept working on the food part, eventually my willpower would grow.

All this focus on food did was take up huge real-estate in my brain. I labeled entire days as "good" and others "bad," depending on what I ate. It wasn't until I moved away for my dietetic internship in New Orleans that things began to change for me. When I got there, I was assigned a dorm without a kitchen. To eat, I had to go to the hospital cafeteria across the street. So I actually felt hungry for meals and began sitting down to eat three balanced meals a day, unlike my constant eating before. I also was faced with indulgent food at every turn. Think fried beignets covered in sugar, white bread slathered in butter, and gumbo made with a rich roux. This kind of food was not the norm in my native California, and to be honest, it kind of scared me.

When a friend pointed out (as I was complaining, of course) that I didn't seem to enjoy eating, I knew she was right. Somewhere along the line, I had lost the enjoyment factor and was eating with my head, not with the intent of satisfying my body. That year, I took a different route with my eating. I still ate nutritious food but began to enjoy non-nutritious items without guilt or overdoing it. My diet became much more balanced, and I really listened to what my body needed. And to my surprise, it didn't want loads of sugar and butter like I feared; it wanted mostly nourishing foods, with some goodies sprinkled in.

I came back to California a new person around food but wasn't quite sure what had happened. My first job was as an outpatient counselor and everyone wanted the food fix. "Just tell me what to eat!" I'd hear, and so I did—and they rarely came back. My next job was at the corporate office at a commercial weight-loss program. Most of the people on the program were return customers. They'd follow the program, lose weight, go back to their life, and gain weight only to come back to lose again. The whole process felt wrong to me so I was off to yet another job. Later in my career, as I began freelance writing, I went back to hospital work and was asked to counsel weight-loss surgery patients. These were people at the end of the road – they had tried every diet and crazy food combination you could think of. I was shocked that none of them understood how their relationship with food affected what and how much they ate.

Throughout the years, I dug into the research, which gave me a solid understanding of what contributed to my previous disordered eating, and how I was able to change my relationship with food. When I became pregnant, I was determined to spare my daughter the suffering around food that could easily happen, which led to my focus on kids and families.

I have written before about teaching kids moderation and managing sweets, but I wanted a comprehensive resource available for parents whom I hated to see struggling. I've read hundreds of journal articles and books, interviewed experts, and have talked on the phone to parents in the thick of it. I wrote this book to take away – and prevent – the needless suffering families encounter every single day. I wrote this book to help parents raise a generation of kids who feel good about eating, their bodies, and their life.

The Mindful Possibilities (and How to Use this Book)

In the best-selling book, *The Art of Possibility,* Roz and Ben Zander encourage readers to embrace life's possibilities based on a powerful idea:

Our premise is that many of the circumstances that seem to block us in our daily lives may only appear to be based on a framework of assumptions we carry with us. Draw a different frame around the same set of circumstances and new pathways come into view. Find the right framework and extraordinary accomplishment becomes an everyday experience.[9]

The framework of assumptions that's been used to manage eating and weight is what I call the Food Framework. It jumps straight to food as the solution by changing, controlling, and monitoring it. But focusing on food without nurturing one's relationship to it is like teaching a child to run before he can even crawl.

In this book, I ask you to put what I call a Mindful Framework on challenges that occur with eating. This is a process of noticing and being aware of what is going on, without rushing to judgment (or food). If you noticed your child constantly going crazy for sweets, for example, instead of reacting you'd ask questions. Does he feel restricted? Is he stressed? What is at the bottom of his relationship with sweets? With a Mindful Framework, you problem-solve more effectively and start treating causes instead of symptoms.

Marci is an example of switching from a Food Framework to a Mindful Framework. When she limited her child's formula, and eventually her food, her daughter went crazy asking to eat all the time. When Marci took a step back, she figured out it was the restriction that was making her child anxious and fixated on food. The answer ended up being about tapping into her daughter's ability to regulate her food intake, a much healthier way to relate to food (more on Marci's story in Principle 2).

I've pinpointed 8 Principles to significantly increase your chances of raising a mindful eater. Although "mindful eater" is typically defined as someone who pays attention while eating, for this book I define a mindful eater as someone who eats for nourishment and enjoyment, uses hunger and fullness to guide eating, and naturally eats in moderation. This is different from a mindless eater who unknowingly eats for other reasons besides nourishment and enjoyment, uses external cues to guide eating, and is more likely to eat in extremes.

Moderation, defined as "avoiding the extremes," is the eating style I believe most parents want for their children. That's because eating in extremes is filled with suffering that goes hand in hand with eating too much food, too little food, or eating in an imbalanced way. As illustrated in Table I.1, the 8 Principles designed to transform your child's relationship with food are the literal gateways to eating well.

Table. I.1: Mindful vs. Food Framework		
Framework	*Type of Eater*	*Results in...*
Mindful Framework: Utilizes the 8 Principles to Find Resolution	Mindful Eater: eats for nourishment and enjoyment, and uses hunger and fullness to guide eating	Eats in Moderation: consumes a variety of food, gets right amount of food for body type, and seeks out nutritious foods
Food Framework: Utilizes a "Food Only" Approach	Mindless Eater: unknowingly eats for non-hunger reasons (boredom, stress, bad feelings), and eats based on external cues	At Risk for Eating in Extremes: consumes too little, too much, or eats in an imbalanced way

The 8 Principles are based on research, expert advice, and insights from families who have been there. Each principle showcases both the Food Framework and Mindful Framework ways of approaching eating challenges, followed by supporting research and stories. This allows you to consider how each has the potential to shape your child's relationship with food, so you can make the best decisions for your family.

Good-to-Know Stuff

This book contains a mix of real-life and inspired-by-real-life stories. The inspired stories are the ones used in the Framework sections, as it was difficult to find families who experienced these two distinct ways of dealing with eating challenges. The rest of the book's stories are based on my private interviews with parents and, in certain cases, the names have been changed to protect people's privacy.

How to Raise a Mindful Eater is not about weight or trying to lose weight. Although I mention weight categories based on BMI (overweight, obese, etc.) and ways to prevent unnecessary weight gain, I never mean to imply that good health is reserved for one size. The approach in this book is about creating the circumstances – a healthy relationship with food – so children can regulate their food intake, which ultimately leads to the appropriate weight for them. This is different than trying to force an ideal size through controlling food intake. That being said, if your child shows accelerated growth that is out of the norm, or if problems have been pestering your child for many years, I highly recommend you seek professional help to get the support you need.

As you read through the 8 Principles, you will find some hit home more than others. Let's say you really struggle with body image concerns addressed in Principle 6 or you want to learn more about teaching nutrition to your child as mentioned in Principle 4. The recommended books and websites at the back of the book can help you learn more from professionals that specialize in that area. Although this book is focused on raising healthy kids, it's for the whole family — and that includes you. Every bit of research points to better success when families partake in health-promoting behaviors together. And if your relationship with food could use some healing, why not heal?

Before digging into the 8 Principles, you need to understand why the Food Framework has such a hold on people despite its obvious shortcomings. There are so many ingrained beliefs about eating, weight, and moderation that need to be addressed. So let's challenge these beliefs to see if they are helping, hurting, or keeping your family stuck.

CHALLENGING THE OLD WAY

"What some call health, if purchased by perpetual anxiety about diet, is no better than tedious disease."
–Alexander Pope

L isa's son was larger than average – with a non-stop appetite since the day he was born. As long as Lisa can remember, she's been limiting his food intake and trying to keep him from gaining too much weight. Her son, now nine, is also very active with competitive soccer and, according to all of his tests, healthy. His pediatrician told Lisa that food and weight will be a struggle for him his entire life.

When I talked to Lisa, I told her that yes, food and weight *can* be a struggle, depending on how you handle it. In fact, struggling is the first sign you're on the wrong track. This is why I had to include this chapter challenging the Food Framework. Because when I talk to parents like Lisa, they kind of get what I am saying, but it's hard to believe and even harder to take action. That's because the Food Framework is so deeply ingrained in us all (health professionals, too), even when it brings about more suffering. This chapter is about prying open this way of approaching eating and looking at it for what it really is.

When you consider the evidence presented here – and the long-term health and well-being of your child – you will see how utilizing a Mindful Framework is hands down the better way to help your child develop a healthy relationship with food.

No one should have to struggle their entire life. No one.

<u>Short-term Fix, Long-term Pain</u>

In a classic World War II study referred to as "The Minnesota Starvation Experiment," 35 normal-weight men were put on a semi-starvation diet for six months. During this period, the men not only lost weight, they became obsessed with food as they collected cookbooks, pinned recipes to bulletin boards, and took part in rituals like adding water to food and eating very slowly.[1] After the study was over, the men were sent home and instructed not to eat too much. Most did, anyway. One participant had his stomach pumped because he couldn't stop himself from eating. Another admitted that no amount of food could cure his craving and vomited on a bus after stuffing himself.[2] How these men related to food before the study (when they ate normally) versus after (feeling starved) was like night and day.

Although this study is an extreme example, it provides a snapshot of what can happen when people feel deprived of food. We see this play out in the research on feeding and children. Researchers Leanne Birch and Jennifer Orlet Fisher first examined the effects of food restriction on children in 1999. When restricted from a palatable food item, preschoolers increased their selection and intake of the target food.[3] In their 2000 study, seven-year-old girls ate a standard lunch followed by free access to snack food afterward. The girls who were restricted at home not only ate more of the snack foods, they felt bad about their eating.[4] In 2013, Brandi Rollins, PhD, Post Doctoral Scholar in Human Development and Family Studies at Penn State designed research to replicate Birch and Fisher's 1999 study, but teased out the effects of restriction based on children's appetite and temperament. The children who found palatable food highly desirable and rated low on inhibitory control ate the most in response to restriction. "Their inability to self-regulate means they go crazy," Rollins said. "Controlling feeding practices only makes this worse." [5]

When researchers follow and observe families, they find that parental restriction is linked to higher weights and poor eating habits in children.[6] In one study that tracked eating in girls from ages five to nine, high levels of restriction at age five predicted what researchers call "eating in the absence of hunger" from ages seven to nine. In addition, the girls who experienced the highest level of restriction at age five were the heaviest at nine.[7]

Dieting, defined by the American Association of Pediatrics (AAP) as "caloric restriction with the goal of weight loss" has been found to increase the risk of both obesity and eating disorders. After reviewing the research, the AAP concluded, "These findings and others suggest that dieting is counterproductive to weight management efforts. Dieting also can predispose to eating disorders."[8] A twin study revealed how going on just one diet increased risk of weight gain by three times. The researchers concluded, "It is now well established that the more people engage in dieting, the more they gain weight."[9]

If these approaches fail long-term, why do we keep using them? Because they work initially. Someone trying to lose weight will shed pounds following a low-calorie meal plan. Removing sweets from the home will keep a child from eating them. This is one of the key ways the Food

Framework keeps us hooked. But as you can see, this initial honeymoon is typically followed by a backfiring effect. When we look deeper, we can see *why* these practices fail long-term despite their initial boost.

It's Psychological and Physiological

When people feel deprived of food, they become hypersensitive to food cues by noticing it everywhere. Then something researchers call "ego depletion" comes into play. This constant resisting of food temptations eventually leads to a depletion of self-control resources, and people give in. "Psychologists have shown clearly that suppression (just saying No) makes ego depletion worse," said Marc Lewis, PhD, neuroscientist and author of *The Biology of Desire*. "Suppressing the impulse gives it more power." This process leads to what researchers call disinhibition: feeling out of control when finally eating a desirable food, the eating behavior most linked to weight gain.[10] The psychological consequences of restricting food intake can be summarized by one of the participants of The Minnesota Starvation Experiment, Harold Blickenstaff:

I don't know many other things in my life that I looked forward to being over with any more than this experiment. And it wasn't so much ... because of the physical discomfort, but because it made food the most important thing in one's life ... food became the one central and only thing really in one's life. And life is pretty dull if that's the only thing. I mean, if you went to a movie, you weren't particularly interested in the love scenes, but you noticed every time they ate and what they ate.[2]

The physiological effects have more to do with the body's natural inclination to fight weight loss in a process called "adaptive thermogenesis." Due to a change in hormones, the body lowers resting metabolic rate (RMR) and increases hunger. Most troubling is the body's compromised ability to become sated at meals. Research suggests these changes occur not just during weight loss, but afterward as well.[11]

A six-year study that included Biggest Loser participants showed that by the end of the competition, RMR decreased by 610 calories. Six years later, when many had regained a considerable amount of weight, metabolic rate was still reduced by 500 calories.[12] Although the decrease in RMR is more extreme with larger amounts of weight loss, studies show it still occurs with more modest losses.[13] This makes weight regain easier with each weight-loss attempt. Then there's "fat overshooting," the body's tendency to regain more fat after intentional weight loss, something that occurs to a greater degree in leaner people. In the rehabilitation part of the Minnesota Starvation Experiment when food was freely offered, intake increased above pre-study levels and stayed that way for weeks, resulting in participants having a higher percentage of fat than when they started.[14]

Both restriction and dieting result in dysregulation, a compromised ability to regulate food intake and recognize hunger and satiety signals. Ironically, this is an important way the Food Framework keeps people hooked. Because when eating gets out of control or weight is regained, people blame themselves or the person struggling, instead of the approach. All the while, people are left to engage in the Food Framework Cycle instead of finding solutions that really work.

Food Framework Cycle

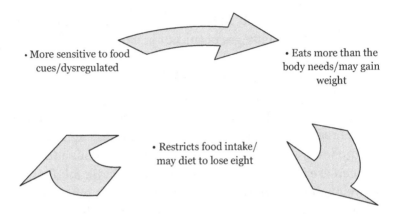

• More sensitive to food cues/dysregulated

• Eats more than the body needs/may gain weight

• Restricts food intake/ may diet to lose eight

<u>Challenging Food Framework's Core Beliefs</u>

I believe that people are starting to reject the idea of dieting and restriction. Yet, this has brought about a situation where people say they aren't dieting or restricting, yet still engage in this type of behavior. For example, it's popular to "eat clean" or "real food" and cut out processed foods like sugar. This can feel a lot like restriction if you (or your child) want to enjoy a cookie with white flour and sugar. And if the change in diet is really done to cut calories for weight loss, that's dieting.

There are three strongly ingrained beliefs that keep the Food Framework alive even when it's being denied on a superficial level. The first is *foods high in sugar, salt, and fat are addictive.* We hear about this constantly in the media, blogs, and popular books. The second is that *overweight and obesity (as defined by BMI) are always bad for health.* This is like background music played daily by the media. And the third is that *the answer to a healthy weight comes down to "healthy eating" and avoiding "bad" foods.* Challenging these core beliefs is how we reject the empty promises of the Food Framework.

Is Food Addiction Real?

I don't know how many times someone has told me either they are or their child is addicted to food. It's no wonder, books and articles on the subject make food addiction seem like a slam dunk. Yet health professionals are far from agreement on it. In fact, there is no classification of an "Overeating Disorder" or an "Addictive Eating Disorder," although there is Binge-Eating Disorder classified under "Feeding and Eating Disorder.[15]" In other words, a clinical diagnosis of food addiction does not exist.

The popular theory being researched and sensationalized in the media is that hyper-palatable foods high in sugar, salt, and fat are addictive like drugs because they share similar reward pathways in the brain. It is described as a neurobiological response to repeated, large intakes of palatable foods resulting in changed reward circuitry in the brain. It starts with the release of "feel-good" dopamine and opioids, followed by over-consumption. As a result, the feel-good response gets blunted, causing people to need even more of the food to get the same reward.

A review article by Dr. Hisham Ziauddeen, senior research associate at Cambridge University, points out the biggest inconsistency – research has not been able to pinpoint an addictive substance like with drugs and alcohol.[16] Is it sugar? Sugar and fat? Sugar, salt, and fat? How much will elicit a response?

"I think the term food addiction sounds like something that many of us may be able to identify with, probably because at some point all of us have been greatly tempted

19

by food that we feel we shouldn't really eat and have often failed to resist the temptation," he said. "However, with food addiction we are really talking about something more severe, an addiction like alcohol or heroin addiction. In my view, the most important fact that people need to bear in mind is that so far we don't really know if such a condition really exists."

The strongest evidence for food addiction has been in animal studies, where researchers use highly palatable foods and very structured feeding environments. The rats do show escalating, binge-like eating behaviors. But when high-sugar or high-fat food is fed in isolation, in addition to the addiction-like behavior (withdrawal symptoms), rats actually self-regulate and do not gain weight. But when fat and sugar are given together in a cafeteria-style diet, they do gain weight but do not exhibit withdrawal symptoms. And reward systems in the brain differ. For example, with drugs, dopamine release stays consistent across various administrations, but with eating, dopamine release stops when the food is no longer novel or the individual is no longer hungry.

Unlike drugs, people need to eat to live. And they overeat for many different reasons such as boredom, negative mood, habit, stress, and as a response to chronic dieting. If people believe that eating is due to something they (or a child) can't control, they may never seek help for the underlying reason that they have issues with food. This is how the concept of food addiction can become a self-fulfilling prophecy. Just hearing the word "addiction" causes people to assume they need to abstain from eating certain foods or to follow a strict diet. Yet, the most effective treatment for people who binge-eat isn't abstinence or restrictive diets, it's cognitive behavioral therapy. Therapists help people change the way they think and relate to food and problem foods are usually brought in so people can learn how to eat those foods without binging.[17]

Self-Fulfilling Prophecy? In a 2015 study in *Appetite,* a group of 60 adults were asked to read an article on food addiction. Half received an article describing it as a myth and the other half read an article explaining how it was real. Fifty-seven percent of those in the "real" condition self-diagnosed themselves as food addicts whereas only 27 percent did in the "myth" condition. When it came to eating indulgent food later, there was more variance in the intake levels among those in the "real" condition.[18]

So people can learn to use food in a compulsive way or not (and if they already learned compulsive patterns they can unlearn them). This book is about helping children relate to food in a healthy way, so they feel in control. In particular, Principle 1 focuses on meal structure so children can build their self-control muscle, Principle 3 is about presenting sweets so they don't get so much attention, and Principle 8 helps kids feel connected and valued, so they are less likely to turn to food.

Once you challenge the belief that addictive foods have all the power, the Food Framework starts looking pretty weak.

Is Weight Directly Tied to Health?

At school, Lily was asked to bring a letter home to give to her mom. When her mom opened it up she read about her daughter being overweight with a BMI of 22. She was outraged! After all, Lily was eleven at the time and 124 pounds with a five-foot-three frame. She also was an active and healthy star volleyball player.[19] The problem is the tendency to directly link weight to health outcomes. BMI is a way to classify weight, not health. And BMI is different for children as it compares values to other children the same age, which put Lily at risk because she weighed more than most other girls her same age, probably due to her muscle mass. BMI's major limitation is it doesn't account for body composition – how much fat and muscle a person has – and emerging research is putting the measure under even more scrutiny.

For instance, a 2013 high profile meta-analysis of more than 100 studies published in the *Journal of American Medical Association* revealed that overweight people (defined as BMI between 25-29) had the lowest mortality rate. Compared to normal weight, only grade two and three obesity (>35 BMI) was significantly associated with mortality.[20] The thing is, this wasn't the first study to show this, just the largest. Other studies show this same U-curve for weight-related health risk meaning risk goes up significantly with a high BMI >35 or low BMI of under 19.[21] The lowest part of the curve is consistently seen with people who are overweight (BMI 25-30). When we look at risk this way, only 14.5 percent of Americans are at risk due to high weights compared to the commonly used 70 percent statistic used for those who are overweight and obese.[22]

There isn't some switch that goes off at higher BMIs either, just increased risk. It is estimated 10-25 percent of people with a BMI >35 have what health professionals call metabolically healthy obesity, meaning they do not have high blood pressure, high cholesterol, and other adverse health outcomes.[23] And there's even a term for people who are metabolically obese at normal weight, meaning they are unhealthy even though weight is normal. People – at any weight – who engage in healthy habits like exercise gain health benefits and lose them when they stop. Linda Bacon, PhD, author of *Body Respect, What Conventional Health Books Get Wrong, Leave Out, or Just Plain Fail to Understand about Weight*, has spearheaded the Health at Every Size (HAES) movement. Her research shows a HAES approach, which focuses on healthy habits over weight outcomes, has positive outcomes in blood pressure, blood lipids like cholesterol, eating habits, exercise, and feelings of well-being.[24]

Although we hear about the endless risks from excess weight, underweight people are actually at greater risk of dying. Researchers looked at 50 studies and found that underweight people were 1.8 times more likely to die than the severely obese who were 1.3 times more likely.[25] "BMI reflects not only body fat, but also muscle mass. If we want to continue to use BMI in health care and public health initiatives, we must realize that a robust and healthy individual is someone who has a reasonable amount of body fat and also sufficient bone and muscle," said lead researcher Dr. Joel Ray in a press release about the study.[26]

So, no, weight is not a direct measure of health, a healthy body is. After evaluating the evidence, the American Academy of Pediatrics recommends pediatricians take the spotlight off of weight: ***"The focus should be on healthy living and healthy habits rather than on weight,"***[8] Someone's weight is just one piece of an intricate health puzzle that includes many factors. We shouldn't throw it out of the equation, but let's stop making it the be-all and end-all of health.

Does a Healthy Weight Boil Down to What a Person Eats?

Any campaign that aims to curb the obesity epidemic – and of course this includes popular diets – almost always focuses on what to eat: getting people to eat less unhealthy foods and more healthy foods. But is it really about getting people to eat the right foods? The idea is healthy foods, like fruits and vegetables, are high in nutrition and filling fiber but low in energy density (calories). If we can get people to eat healthy, then obesity will reverse itself.

Overall, studies that look into the effect of fruits and vegetables on weight are not impressive. One review made the following conclusion: "On the basis of the current evidence, recommending increased fruit and vegetable consumption to treat or prevent obesity without explicitly combining this approach with efforts to reduce intake of other energy sources is unwarranted."[27] Of course fruits and vegetables are beneficial to health regardless of weight. But the key to avoiding unnecessary weight gain has more to do with *how* people eat than *what* they eat. It makes more sense to create circumstances that encourage optimal food regulation. People who don't regulate their food intake are more likely to eat more or less than their bodies need.

There are different ways scientists test food regulation, but the most common is to feed what they call a "preload," followed by free access to food. Then researchers see how well people adjust their intake, which can happen over the course of a day or more (especially for children). When adjustments in consumption aren't made after eating, food regulation may be limited. Research suggests that infants and young children have better food-regulation skills than older children and adults.[28] The Food Framework tells us it's because of the type of food we have available today but in the 1950s when obesity wasn't an epidemic, meat, butter, sugary drinks, bread, and dessert were regular visitors at the family table. Let's examine the five key factors that are most likely behind poor food regulation and the food choices people make:

Not enough sleep

Research suggests that about one-third of working adults and 75 percent of adolescents (by 12th grade) get insufficient sleep.[28,29] Inadequate sleep has repeatedly been linked to higher calorie intake and found to produce a more robust appetite for empty-calorie foods high in sugar and fat.[30]

Trouble managing modern-day stress

Stress has been on the rise but modern stress is different because of its psychological basis. According to The American Institute of Stress:

...the nature of stress for modern man is not an occasional confrontation with a saber-toothed tiger or a hostile warrior but rather a host of emotional threats like getting stuck in traffic and fights with customers, co-workers, or family members, that often occur several times a day. Unfortunately, our bodies still react with these same, archaic fight or flight responses that are now not only not useful but potentially damaging.[31]

Excess stress is associated with increased intake of energy-dense foods and overall food intake. It also can adversely affect sleep.[32]

Inactivity

Physical activity has been on the decline – at work, home and during travelling – for decades. In 1960, for instance, 67 percent of trips to work used cars, but this jumped to 88 percent in 2000. Forty percent of children rode their bike to school in 1969, but this dipped to only 13 percent in 2001.[33] People who are inactive gain more weight over time than those who aren't. Not only that, being sedentary compromises the body's ability to regulate food. Research also shows that physical activity promotes consumption of nutritious foods like fruits and vegetables.[34]

Eating in the absence of hunger

Snacking has been on the rise for decades but it's not just snacking that's problematic — it's eating when not hungry. According to a Mintel survey that included Millennials — the first generation to grow up with the snacking culture — 27 percent said they snack due to boredom and 17 percent said they snack when stressed.[35] In another survey, 34 percent of adults said they have acquired the habit of overeating while stressed, and teens responded at an even higher 37 percent.[36] Distracted eating, linked to compromised food regulation, has become more common with advances in technology as people eat while checking their computer, watching TV, or while playing video games.[37]

Restriction and diets for weight loss

Half of adults want to reduce their weight and believe restricting portion size and reduced/low-calorie products are the way to get there.[38] Half of adolescent girls and a third of adolescent boys have utilized unhealthy weight-control behaviors to control their weight.[39] As stated earlier, restriction and diets can eventually backfire in terms of food choice and regulation, and don't address the underlying causes of weight gain or poor eating.

The Old Way...

Wait until weight is a problem and then work to "get" to a healthy weight by controlling food.

The New (Better) Way...

Support all children (from day one) in growing into a weight that is right for them by creating the circumstances for optimal food regulation. When eating problems arise — at any age — look to root causes to find answers.

The Food Framework loves to target food, but isn't it time we pay attention to what is actually impeding food regulation and food choice in the first place? The good news is there is a better way to approach eating that is gaining some serious steam.

The Intuitive Eating Revolution

Even back in the 1980s when counting calories was all the rage, dietitians Evelyn Tribole and Elyse Resch were wary about giving weight-loss advice, especially in the form of diets. Being in private practice they found that the doctors kept referring patients for weight loss so they created meal plans to help their clients lose weight. They did so gently, never calling these plans diets, and they encouraged people to include all foods, albeit sensibly. Their clients did lose weight but when they heard back from them at a later date, they gained it back and felt terrible, blaming themselves.

Eventually, the two teamed up to create a new paradigm centered on a very different approach to food. At the time, programs with a no-diet focus were already gaining momentum, but they didn't like the idea of throwing nutrition out the window, as many of these programs did. This led to their well-known intuitive eating approach first brought to the public in the first edition of *Intuitive Eating* in 1995.[40] On their website, Tribole and Resch define intuitive eating this way:

...an approach that teaches you how to create a healthy relationship with your food, mind, and body — where you ultimately become the expert of your own body. You learn how to distinguish between physical and emotional feelings, and gain a sense of body wisdom.[41]

The approach has ten principles to guide individuals, with these three key factors driving them:

1) Unconditional permission to eat
2) Eating for physical rather than emotional reasons
3) Relying on internal cues (hunger and fullness) to guide eating

Although this concept was born out of the need to help adults, a key component of Intuitive eating is to *"...be able to ultimately return to your inborn Intuitive Eater..."* The idea is that we are all born with these innate skills but they are driven out of us in the modern food culture. This book helps you protect this inborn ability in your child, and if your child's gotten off track, return them back to this state. The three key domains that encompass Intuitive Eating – and how they relate to feeding children – are described in Table 1.1.

Table 1.1: Intuitive Eating and Feeding Children

IE Domains	What it is	Why?	How it Relates to Feeding Children
Unconditional permission to eat	No food is forbidden or off limits	Less likely to overindulge and fixate on food. Chooses nutritious food willingly	Neutral presentation of a variety of food instead of labeling them good or bad (Principles 3 and 4)
Eating for physical rather than emotional reasons	Eat for hunger and enjoyment instead of boredom, anxiety, stress or habit (car, TV, night)	Less binge-eating and eating in the absence of hunger	Structured meals at the table (Principle 1)
Relying on internal cues of hunger and fullness to guide eating	Trusting internal cues to decide how much to eat	Aids food regulation so people get the right amount of food for their body type	Tune into hunger and satiety cues by paying attention (Principle 2)

The Research Behind Intuitive Eating

In the beginning, the research used to support intuitive eating focused on what didn't work (dieting and restriction). In 2006, Tracy Tylka, PhD, created an intuitive eating scale (IE scale) to spearhead research in this area.[42] Just a decade later, there are more than 40 studies published, and here's what the research reveals:

Weight

Studies consistently show that people who score high on the IE scale have lower BMIs compared to those who don't. This shows a link, and not cause and effect, but research suggests intuitive eating plays a protective role when it comes to unnecessary weight gain.[43]

Food attitudes and general well-being

Studies show intuitive eaters are less likely to participate in unhealthy weight control practices. In one study, young adults who trusted their body in regards to hunger and fullness had a lower risk of disordered eating than those who didn't.[44] And the intuitive eating young women were less likely to diet and binge eat. Studies also show that intuitive eaters report higher self-esteem, improved life satisfaction, positive coping skills, and more food enjoyment compared to non-intuitive eaters.

Healthy behaviors and body satisfaction

People who score higher on the IE scale report a more diverse diet, more physical activity, and a positive body image.[43]

Other Internal Approaches to Eating

Other internal approaches to eating have supportive research as well. Mindful eating, the process of paying attention at meals without judgment, has been effective in a number of studies. According to one review on mindful eating interventions, 92 percent of the studies show reductions in binge-eating episodes, 63 percent show improvements in emotional eating, 67 percent report improvements in external eating and 90 percent of the studies that had weight as an outcome showed people either maintained or lost weight.[45]

Another similar eating concept is Ellyn Satter's eating competence. According to Satter, competent eaters have a positive and relaxed attitude about eating, are internally motivated to choose nutritious foods, use internal cues of hunger and fullness to guide eating, and plan and structure eating at predictable times throughout the day. Research suggests that those who score high on eating competence eat healthier diets, have similar or lower BMIs, are more active, sleep better, have better lab tests, and do a better job feeding their children than those who don't.[46]

These internal approaches to eating don't focus on food rules at all. Instead, they lay the groundwork for a healthy relationship with food, which is a better way to improve eating and health in today's world.

From Struggle to Answers

Lisa, introduced in the beginning of the chapter, was told her son would struggle with eating and weight his whole life. No doubt, the Food Framework sets this up perfectly. Those three ingrained beliefs got her. Fearing food addiction, she tried to keep simple carbs out of his reach, which was impossible 24/7. She worried he wouldn't be healthy at a higher weight so she limited how much he ate, which of course only made him want to eat more. And she spent many meals trying to get him to eat healthy (not go for the starchy food first, etc.), something that never seemed to make him want to choose nutritious items. All of these controlling practices only made both her and her son feel less in control when it came to food and his body. It produced the Food Framework Cycle that keeps so many families stuck.

Now Lisa is curious about a different way, and I hope you are too. And it's not just a theory, it has a growing body of research to support it. Instead of fearing food addiction, you will learn how to help your child relate to food in healthy ways. Instead of focusing on weight, you will create the circumstances for optimal food regulation which includes an internal approach to eating. And instead of always harping on what your child should eat, you'll help him come to truly value healthy habits.

Most books of this nature start and stop with the internal approach to eating, but I fear this isn't enough, especially when raising children. A Mindful Framework will not only help you initiate an internal approach to eating, but sustain it. In other words, there's a lot that can stand in your way of success, luring you back into the Food Framework. I talk to parents all the time who started off trusting children with food but get tripped up when they become picky, snack non-stop, or seem out of control with sweets. Seeing eating through a Mindful Framework helps you work through these barriers so you can keep your child's relationship with food intact as they work their way up to adulthood.

This is why the 8 Principles target four key areas. The first is establishing an internal approach to eating in the first place. The next three deal with barriers that can get in the way like your child's food preferences, how they come to view their body, and managing stress. These are the things most people don't think about because they aren't specifically about food. Whether you're here to prevent eating problems or find solutions (or likely both), these principles touch on the most likely contributors.

1) *Internal Approaches to Eating:* Principles 1 and 2 provide guidance on structuring meals, setting limits, eating based on internal cues of hunger and fullness, and paying attention while eating.
2) *Balance Food for Nourishment and Enjoyment:* Principles 3, 4 and 5 help you find lasting ways to make nutrition rewarding, sweets less desirable, and eating well a pleasurable experience.
3) *Body Appreciation and Self-care:* Principles 6 and 7 give you the tools you need to teach your child how to appreciate her body, develop and maintain a positive body image, and learn the art of self-regulation.
4) *Mental and Emotional Happiness:* Principles 7 and 8 provide guidance on identifying and managing stressors, processing difficult emotions, and making family connection a priority.

Once you commit and master the 8 Principles, your family will be set free from the chains of the Food Framework. It will feel good to finally get answers and feel in control of food instead of the other way around. A healthier and happier life awaits.

THE 8 PRINCIPLES

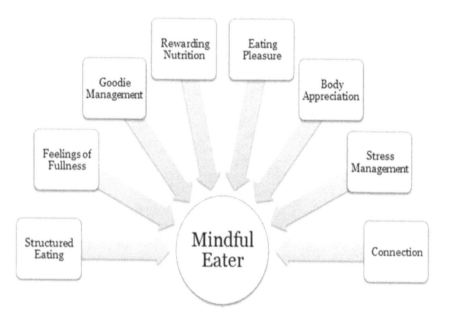

PRINCIPLE 1

PLAN, PRIORITIZE, AND STRUCTURE MEALS

"I value self-discipline, but creating systems that make it next to impossible to misbehave is more reliable than self-control." –Tim Ferriss

Charlotte's five-year-old daughter, Kelly, ate more than she did. When Charlotte contacted me, she didn't know what to do. She was concerned for her daughter's health as her weight was creeping up. "She has been like this for about the past two years, and I am curious if there is any reason that she would feel this way," she said. "What can I do to stop her from eating too much?" Charlotte described how after meals her daughter comes back ten minutes later asking for a snack. "If her wish isn't granted, she screams and cries until she gets some sort of snack or food."

When I ask her if she gives into her daughter's request she said she "tries not to." Soon, I discover Kelly has been going into the cupboards for food since she was two.

Charlotte nags her daughter not to touch the junk that her husband brings home, but that rarely works. Although it seems like the child's eating is the problem, it's actually the lack of enforced limits the child is pushing up against.

Planning, prioritizing, and structuring meals is the best place to start for anyone aiming to raise a mindful eater. After all, this was how people successfully ate before snacking, grazing, and eating on the go became a national pastime. In addition, kids with too much freedom around the *what, when* and *where* of eating simply don't eat as well. It can take real effort to get started, especially when you have a spirited child like Kelly. Yet once you get this important part of feeding down and stay consistent, you will never want to go back to how things were before. Trust me on this!

First, let's consider why the Food Framework way of dealing with hunger management is limited and may create even more problems.

The Food Framework – Taming Hunger with Healthy Food

Angela's daughter, Casey, was always hungry. She was a good eater for the most part, ate quite a bit of nutritious foods, but it was her appetite that worried Angela. Casey was also larger than average, and obesity ran in their family, adding to the concern. Angela worked hard to have healthy choices available when Casey declared her hunger. Of course, they had snack-type food too, like crackers and pretzels, but she always tried to lead Casey to healthy choices. She also made Casey wait sometimes when she asked for food, asking her to play first and if she was still hungry in a bit, she could eat. Angela felt exhausted trying to tame her daughter's appetite and satisfy her with healthy foods.

Yet no amount of eating healthy stopped the constant hunger issue. The truth was Casey was disconnecting to her feelings of hunger and fullness due to the free flow of food allowed. While not intentional, saying "I'm hungry" was her way of getting food when she wanted it. She was learning to eat when bored, when doing homework, and when she felt overwhelmed. She was developing a relationship with food where eating was becoming associated with activities and feelings, instead of hunger and enjoyment.

The Problem with Permissive Feeding

I like to use the example of a seesaw to describe how parents feed their kids and the energy it takes. There's what I call Control Feeding, which is like pushing yourself up on the seesaw. That's because it takes a lot of energy to control and regulate a child's eating. Permissive Feeding is like going down when seesawing by just pulling your feet up and falling. This is when you let children do what they want, saying yes, or giving in. From my experience, parents often find themselves seesawing between Control and Permissive feeding. When controlling a child's food intake becomes too difficult to maintain, then parents put their feet up (or hands) and go down. This constant up and down takes a lot of energy for parents and it sends mixed signals to children.

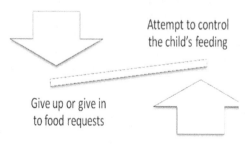

Attempt to control
the child's feeding

Give up or give in
to food requests

Permissive and Control Feeding are associated with higher child BMI, negative health outcomes, and increased risk of obesity.[1] Permissive Feeding is particularly problematic because it doesn't set up boundaries for children allowing them to strengthen their self-control muscle. If they want a food, they can have it anytime. If they are just slightly hungry, they get food the instant they say so. They can much more easily lose track of hunger and fullness, eating too much or too little. Parents may not always be aware of how much kids are eating between meals and may also push them to eat come dinnertime, which negatively affects their ability to regulate food.

Without some limits and understanding of when and where to eat, children are more likely to associate eating with activities rather than hunger. In one study, preschool children associated food with almost a quarter of their daily activities.[2] And it's no wonder, snacking is on the rise and takes up almost one-third of daily calories. There has also been an increase in salty snacks and candy as prime food choices, even though desserts and sweetened beverages remain the major sources of calories from snacks.[3] We also know the more children accumulate eating behaviors like skipping breakfast, snacking between meals, and watching TV while eating, the higher their weights are likely to be.[4]

So children are not only snacking more, making food associations, and eating mindlessly, they're also choosing food that is low in nutrition. The Food Framework tells us it's about removing the bad food and replacing it with healthy items. But it's really about the missing system (meal structure) and making sure the feeding responsibility of parents and child is where it needs to be.

Crossing the Division of Responsibility

When feeding gets off track there's a simple way to determine where the problem lies. It's based on international feeding expert Ellyn Satter's Division of Responsibility, which defines two different feeding/eating responsibilities for parents and children. It's the parent's job to decide the *what, when* and *where* of feeding, and it's the child's job to decide the *whether* and *how much* of eating.[5]

Satter's Division of Responsibility	
Parent's Job	*Child's Job*
• Decide what to serve while considering child's food preferences	• Decide what to eat from what is served at meal or snack time
• Decide when the family eats and where, such as the kitchen table	• Decide how much to eat based on feelings of hunger and fullness

When there are problems with feeding, it usually occurs because parent, or child, is crossing the Division of Responsibility. For example, when children are allowed to freely get food and eat wherever they like, they are taking over all three parts of a parent's job: what to eat, when to eat, and where. Permissive feeding is mostly about children taking over their parents' job, where Control Feeding, discussed in the next chapter, is about parents taking over the child's job of deciding what and how much to eat from what is offered.

Both the stories presented with Kelly and Casey show that these kids were taking over the parent's job of when to eat. Although one was going directly to the cabinets, and the other was asking, they both were crossing the Division of Responsibility. Feeding on demand works great for breast and formula feeding but as kids get past age three, they become more sensitive to environmental cues of eating. No doubt, certain kids may be fine waiting until they are hungry to eat but it can be a slippery slope. As you will see, structure with eating helps children learn how to effectively manage their hunger, develop self-control, and avoid the pitfalls of mindless eating.

The Mindful Framework – A Regular Rhythm of Meals and Snacks

When Angela adopted a Mindful Framework, she could see that structuring meals and snacks was key to helping her daughter. First, she let her daughter Casey know that things would be changing and there would be no eating between planned meals and snacks, and that they will be eaten at the table. She asked Casey for input on foods she'd like to see so she could include those at meals and snacks periodically. She also started doing a better job of planning meals and snacks every week so she didn't have to constantly think about what to eat. She developed a rotation for breakfasts and snacks and had dinner planned for the whole week.

The first week was the toughest as Casey still asked for food in between meals. But Angela gently reminded her when the next eating occasion would be and encouraged her to do other activities. Once Casey got accustomed to their rhythm of eating, she seemed more satisfied with meals and snacks and then stopped asking for food. Best of all, she was figuring out other things to do besides eat, like read or jump on the trampoline. She had a few more meltdowns, but Angela realized this was because she was learning how to manage uncomfortable feelings without running to food. She also ate better overall with a hearty appetite at mealtime.

Planning meals ended up really helping Angela, too. She no longer spent a good portion of her day thinking about what to serve, or trying to curb her child's hunger. Her week flowed much more easily and everyone seemed happier. The best part is she stopped worrying about Casey's eating and future weight. She realized her daughter was developing a healthy relationship with food and could indeed be satisfied and get the right amount of food for her body.

Benefits of Meal Structure (and a Moderate Feeding Style)

Structuring meals and snacks at a designated place, without in-between meal eating, is incredibly valuable. Children learn to view food as a priority, and are more likely to become mindful eaters. With a regular rhythm of meals and snacks, they feel secure about food. They don't associate food with everyday activities because most meals and snacks are eaten in a designated place, like the kitchen table. Best of all, children are able to tune into their hunger and get the right amount of food for their body type.

Unlike Permissive and Control Feeding Styles, a Moderate Feeding Style makes this happen by setting clear limits in a warm and responsive way. It's staying true to Satter's Division of Responsibility without the child or parent doing the wrong job. If we go back to the seesaw, instead of going up and down, with Moderate Feeding, parent and child just peacefully sit on the seesaw. This takes the least amount of energy and is the perfect balance between Control and Permissive Feeding. This style of feeding has been linked to higher fruit and vegetable intake and has been found to be protective against obesity.[1] Researchers believe it's the structure and limits around food, something they term "structure-based feeding," that enhances self-control and improves eating habits. This is adopted from the parenting literature showing that structure in the home is linked to better self-discipline in children.[6]

Dr. Laura Markham, author of *Peaceful Parent, Happy Kids* and creator of the online site Aha Parenting, explains the benefits this way:

So every time your child chooses to shift gears from what she wants to do, to follow your lead, she practices regulating her impulses. She's building self-discipline muscle. (Or actually, neural pathways. But like muscle, these neural pathways get stronger with use, so you can think of it as building a stronger brain that's capable of harder work.). Permissive parenting doesn't help kids develop self-discipline because it doesn't ask them to exercise self-control in pursuit of their larger goal. [7]

Researchers set out to discover what type of meal routines were linked to healthier eating in college students. Those who ate nutrient-rich diets were more likely to regularly prepare meals and eat breakfast and dinner. Unhealthy eating habits were linked to eating on the run, eating while engaging in other activities (like checking your phone), and purchasing food on campus. The authors of the study recommend that nutrition messages should include advice on how to structure meals in addition to dietary advice.[8] Here's the thing – preparing and sharing meals leads to more nutritious eating, not the other way around. This is one thing that parents have great control over – *how* their families eat. Structuring balanced meals at the table, making them enjoyable, and encouraging kids to listen to hunger and fullness is powerful stuff.

But sometimes that means you have to say "no."

A Better Way to Say No to Food

The secret to setting limits is to not be insensitive to what your child wants and not bark orders; it's to say "no" more effectively – and with a large dose of empathy. Consider these two ways of saying no to a child's food request:

- "For the fourth time I told you no. PLEASE don't ask me again. No cookies!"
- "I know you want cookies with your friend, but it's too close to dinnertime, and I don't want to spoil your appetite. Plus, we're having your favorite pudding for dessert tonight."

Which limit do you think the child will respond better to? The second one, of course. Why? Because it not only shows empathy but also explains the why behind the decision. When parents constantly say no without explaining the *why* behind it and *when* the child will get the item (or something similar), children are left frustrated and wanting more. But when we add some context, it not only softens the blow, it teaches children about balanced choices.

Dr. Laura Markham explains why empathy and understanding is so essential to the process of setting limits:

Because your child is less likely to struggle against the limit. She may not like your limit, but she feels your understanding and compassion. She knows you're on her side. So she chooses to stop fighting for what she wants, so she can have something she wants more – to stay lovingly connected to you. She chooses to regulate her own impulses. She accepts your limit, and even internalizes it – makes it her own.[7]

The secret to Moderate Feeding is enforcing structure with a good dose of compassion and understanding. This mix helps kids listen better and do what we want, even when they don't want to. The next part of the process is figuring out how many times a day your child needs to eat.

Figuring Out Mealtimes

When planning meals and snacks, you'll first have to consider your child's size and age. An adult's stomach is about the size of a football while a toddler's is the size of his fist. This is why newborns eat every one-to-three hours around the clock, and as their stomachs grow, they can go longer and eventually stop the night feeds.

By one year, most children are eating about six times per day, with the last meal typically consisting of milk or a breastfeeding session. Toddlers tend to eat every two-to-three hours (five or six meals) while preschoolers may be able to go three, maybe even four hours between meals. Sample meal plans, like those in the American Academy of Pediatrics Pediatric Nutrition Handbook, recommend three main meals and two in-between meal snacks for the average toddler/preschooler.[9]

By school age, children can move to a "three meal and one afternoon snack" routine, but timing of breakfast and lunch matter. For example, a child that starts school early (7:30), meaning breakfast is at seven or earlier, who doesn't have lunch until 12:30, would need something in between.

Understanding your child's growth and development, something my coauthor and I go into great detail about in *Fearless Feeding,* is key to deciding how often to offer food.[10] As said earlier, younger children need to be offered food more frequently, but they should be the ones to choose whether to eat or not. With growth spurts and changing appetites, parents need to remember that food intake will vary at meals. Here are some basic guidelines to keep in mind:

Toddler: 5–6 times per day (3 meals and 2–3 snacks)
Preschooler: 5 times per day (3 meals and 2 snacks)
School Age: 4–5 times per day (3 meals and 1–2 snacks)

Of course every child will be different. When my son was three years old, for instance, he probably would've done fine eating four times a day because he was such a big breakfast eater and never seemed hungry for his mid-morning snack. But when my daughter was three, she barely ate at meals (she went three weeks one time eating only one bite at breakfast!), and frequent meals were a must. Not only is each child different, but your child is constantly changing. That's childhood for you!

Structure-Based Feeding (Before and After)

Once you decide how many times to feed your child, you can let him know the plan. Explain the changes to him (unless he is too young to understand) and how you will be in charge of what, when, and where food is offered while considering his preferences. But he gets to decide how much and whether or not to eat. Most of all, be clear that there is no eating between meals and snacks.

Structure-based feeding is more like a flexible routine than a strict eating schedule. If it's the weekend and my kids eat a big or late breakfast, I will bring a light snack or just move lunch up earlier. When we go to parties, this is all thrown out the window as my kids can choose what to eat like anyone at the party (they often graze). These are exceptions, not the rule. You never want this routine to become a negative, so always monitor how things are going. Let's look at some before and after examples of how it works.

School day (before)

Eight-year-old Joey is used to getting up and picking his breakfast, which typically is cereal and milk. He then goes to sit at the table and eats while on his tablet. His mom packs a lunch and snack that he has at school, but when he gets home, he goes straight to the kitchen and pulls out the best stuff he can find – Doritos. He usually eats on the chair in his room while playing on his tablet again. Some days this constant snacking goes on for over an hour, and he often isn't hungry for dinner.

School day (after)

Joey's mom creates a weekly rotation for breakfast and lets him know about it. Tuesdays and Fridays are cereal days so he can pick his cereal, but he also needs to include a fruit or smoothie. The other days include items like egg sandwiches and yogurt with fruit. He also needs to eat at the table without playing with his tablet. When he gets home from school, a balanced snack is also planned (he's learning how to make these, too) and he eats at the table before doing anything else. His mom makes sure he stops eating at least two hours before dinner, allowing him to gain back an appetite.

Lazy weekend (before)

A couple with young children are good at planning breakfast and dinner on weekends but what's eaten in between is anybody's guess. The kids are in and out of the kitchen grazing on snacks or are constantly reaching for snacks when they are out. Although they bring fruit and other real food, the kids always want the crackers, goldfish, and pretzels. They are always asking to eat these foods in the car.

Lazy weekend (after)

The parents start planning lunches on the weekend, one at home, and one out. The kids are no longer allowed to graze all day when at home or in the car. They typically have the mid-morning snack while they are out and the other at home in the afternoon, although sometimes these are skipped if breakfast or lunch is late. The parents provide more variety at snack time, too. Sometimes it's fruit and cheese; other times nuts and yogurt; and sometimes Goldfish crackers.

Outside food (before)

In one family, the mom has a hard time saying no, so her kids are always having the cookie at the store, lollipops, or donuts after church. In another family, the mom is always saying no, so the kids rarely get to have treats outside of home and start to focus on them more.

Outside food (after)

Instead of always saying yes or no, use the structure of meals to guide your answer to food requests. If it's close to snack time, and you are out and about and a snack is offered, then a yes may be in order. If your child hasn't had something sweet – and wants something sweet that is offered – it may also be a yes or a choice between now or later. But if it's close to mealtime and your child wants the free cookie at the store, then that's a no because it's too close to mealtime. Or if you had unexpected ice cream after lunch and your child asks about dessert, that's a likely no and it helps to remind her she had something sweet earlier.

Still hungry between meals

There are times kids get extra hungry between meals, especially during growth spurts. You can try the fruit strategy my coauthor and I detail in *Fearless Feeding*. For example, you might say something like, "I know you're hungry, but I don't want to spoil your appetite for dinner, which is only 30 minutes away. How about a piece of fruit to tide you over?" Raw veggies with dip also is a great way to tide over kids until dinner without wrecking their appetite.

Plan, Prioritize and Structure Meals Summary

Planning, prioritizing and structuring meals is your main job. Offering children a variety of food in a structured, empathetic, and consistent way, helps build their self-discipline muscle. Here are the main points of Principle 1 to keep in mind moving forward:

1) Every week plan breakfasts, lunches, dinners, and snacks. Post on the fridge and review with children; consider changes based on their input.
2) If kids are used to a loose feeding schedule, explain clearly to them how things are going to change. Review Satter's Division of Responsibility, explaining that it's your job to pick what to eat, when to eat it, and where but they get to decide how much and whether or not to eat it.
3) Let children know that you decide what is for meals but you want their input. School-aged children can start making some meals and snacks, but it's important they do it with guidance from parents.
4) Decide how many times to eat meals and snacks. Three meals and two snacks is typical, but that depends on needs, and different children have different needs.
5) Designate a place to eat, like the kitchen table. Limit eating while watching TV, playing video games, or in the car to occasional occurrences.
6) Enforce these limits with understanding and empathy. When saying no to food requests be sure to explain the why, so kids also learn about the ins and outs of balanced eating.

When kids understand there are certain times for eating, they stop asking for food and learn to manage their hunger. It brings a nice peace and rhythm to eating, your home, and life. And it's the first and very vital step to raising a mindful eater.

Next, helping kids listen to their bodies and pay attention while eating.

PRINCIPLE 2

ALLOW HUNGER AND FULLNESS TO GUIDE EATING

"When I first realized how simple it was to end the compulsion with food – eat what your body wants when you're hungry, stop when you've had enough – I felt as if I had popped out of life as I knew it and suddenly found myself in another galaxy."
–Geneen Roth

Marci, introduced early in the book, was terrified to allow her daughter to decide how much to eat from what she served. No doubt, she went a bit crazy at first, but when she started leaving food on her plate and no longer thought about food 24/7, Marci knew it was working.

She admits that it's a long process and challenges still come up. "There are going to be different situations, and each kid is going to respond differently," she said. "There are the standard guidelines, but you need to be willing to go back to the drawing board when things aren't working."

Marci admitted it was tempting to panic and stop. Yet she always came back to the same thing – her child's relationship with food. Mealtimes had become so stressful, like noticing how much butter and syrup on a pancake her daughter took. Now, she focuses on her daughter. It's such a relief!

One of the greatest gifts you can give your child is the ability to allow hunger and fullness to guide their eating. It sounds easy, but in today's world it's not, especially when you have a big or small eater that is big or small in size. But as you will see, it's the next essential step to raising a mindful eater.

The Food Framework – Controlling How Much

Debbie enjoyed feeding her son, Zack, when he was a baby. He ate almost everything and this continued on (more or less) until he was three. Then, he started picking at food and refusing many of the healthy items he had eaten before. Zack was also thin, something that didn't bother Debbie when he was eating a lot, but she worried he wasn't getting enough to eat. She started asking him to take more bites and even used dessert as a reward for eating. When he did finish something on his own, she was sure to praise him. As he entered school, he ate more on his own, and she felt relieved.

As Zack got older, Debbie noticed he always ate a lot and still would ask for a second portion of dessert. His weight started climbing, and even though the pediatrician wasn't concerned (BMI normal even though growing off his regular curve), something didn't seem right. So Debbie started limiting sweets and keeping him to one hearty portion at dinner. He started to ask for food all the time, and she constantly battled him to eat less. Then, she found out he was sneaking goodies at school and lying about how much he ate at a friend's house.

Zack had become disconnected to his internal cues of hunger and fullness. Early on, he learned to clean his plate regardless of how he was feeling. As he got older and his appetite increased, he found it hard to stop eating. The restrictions only caused him to be more focused on food, until it became all he could think about.

The Problem with Control Feeding

For most of human history, food was scarce, so children had to eat when food was available. The difference today is food is not scarce, it's everywhere. Yet many parents still use this strategy of making sure kids eat enough. According to one study, 85 percent of parents of young children try to get them to eat more with rewards, praise, and encouragement.[1] Another study showed that half of parents of adolescents ask children to clean their plates.[2]

Pressuring kids to eat is linked to eating based on external cues, eating for emotional reasons, and disordered eating.[3] In one study, college students who remember being picky as kids reported if their parents exerted pressure or not. Picky eating by itself was not linked to eating problems in young adulthood. It was only when pressure was combined with picky eating that the students reported lower intuitive eating and more disordered eating symptoms.[4]

Then there's restriction, the most common feeding strategy utilized for kids perceived as having a weight problem. We've talked about the consequences of restriction, such as eating when not hungry and becoming more sensitive to food cues. Often, pressure and restriction are used together. Attempting to get children to eat more healthy food, for example, while restricting them from unhealthy items. Experts believe that all this noise at mealtime works to override kids' internal cues of eating until they get to the point they stop listening to their bodies.

In the last principle, we touched on the problem that occurs when kids cross Satter's Division of Responsibility by taking over their parents' job of deciding when to eat and sometimes what and where. Control Feeding is when parents take over the child's job of deciding what to eat and how much. This is what happened with Zack. Except for when he was a baby, he had always been told how much to eat, without any regard to feelings of fullness.

Who Knows Best?

When children are born, there's a lot they don't know and need to learn. They don't know how to put together a balanced meal or have the wherewithal to decide to sit in a designated place to eat, as mentioned in the last principle. They also don't know how to cook or set a table, all things parents teach over time.

But children know when they've had enough or when they are hungry for more. As mentioned in the beginning of the book, we are all born intuitive eaters unless there is an underlying issue. Children also know how food tastes and feels in their mouth. If they don't like the texture or taste of a food, they will spit it out. But there's something neither child nor parent knows – the plan for their body. Maybe they are going to be really tall or muscular, all unknowns that can affect appetite. Parents trying to control these in-born factors may start to see even more eating problems crop up. In one study, children whose parents used food rewards and restriction with their child at three-to five-years old had a child significantly more likely to eat for emotional reasons at five-to seven-years old.[5] The Food Framework tells us it's because the kids simply don't know when to stop eating, but we know better after challenging this limiting way of seeing food.

You are certainly not a bad parent if you use control, or have used it, at the table. Most of us do because controlling one's eating (via the Food Framework) is the norm of society. The problem is, this is the wrong tool to use. Instead, you can work to greatly influence your child by taking control of the right things, which is illustrated in Table P2.1, and the rest of this chapter (and book).

Table P2.1: Take Control of the Right Things	
Can't control...	*But you can...*
High appetite by giving less food	• Serve filling foods/reliable meals • Help child tune in at meals • Check non-food factors (Principles 6-8)
Slow rate of food acceptance by forcing food or pressuring a child to eat	• Up food exposure • Teach child about different foods • Be a role model

The good news is if you've gotten off track, it's never too late to put children back in touch with their bodies. And it starts with a Mindful Framework.

The Mindful Framework – Helping a Child Recognize Hunger & Fullness

When Debbie noticed Zack eat more and more without regard to being full, she knew something wasn't right. What really did it for her was his reaction to her cutting him off – he didn't like it! Using a Mindful Framework, she realized that getting her son to eat more and using dessert as a reward were mistakes. Now that he was getting hungrier playing sports and being exposed to more food, he ate for external reasons – food on the plate, a goodie in sight, and anytime he saw food!

Deciding to make a change was not easy as her son was almost ten now. But she sat him down and explained where she went wrong and why she wanted things to change. He told her he does know hunger and fullness, but she said she wanted to focus on it more, anyway. Since she had been restricting him, when he was allowed to eat as much as he wanted, he overate for about a week. But she also stopped dessert after every dinner, something they had done since he was little. He didn't like it but she planned out days he'd have sweets for snack time and the occasional dinner. When he wanted more food, she'd give it to him but also reminded him to tune in, and after about a month she noticed a difference in him.

She also talked about how different foods make you full and provide lasting energy, and that interested him. They started experimenting with cooking together. As a result, he added some new foods such as beans, hearty salads, and a sandwich served with soup instead of chips. He liked how these foods helped him feel full, and gave him energy for his active life. He gradually made the switch from being an external eater to someone who used internal cues to guide

58

his eating.

Trust vs. Control

When I asked researcher Tracy Tylka the biggest myth about intuitive eating, she said "That once individuals begin to eat intuitively, they will completely lose control and eat everything (high in sugar, high in fat) in sight and gain a bunch of weight, and that people cannot trust their internal hunger and satiety cues and have to rely on external rules to govern eating."

When Marci finally committed to a trust model of feeding, her biggest fear was not realized. Her child's weight actually went down a bit, although she stayed larger than average, which was her natural frame. Yet the truth is she stopped thinking about her daughter's weight after seeing how well she could regulate her food intake. Most importantly, Marci explained, is that her daughter likes herself and is healthy. Her advice for moms is "It's just a good thing and it works. You just have to trust it's going to work. If you only do it halfway you'll never get to the point where they can trust their bodies."

A good place to start is making your kitchen table reflect this newfound trust. This can be done by serving meals family style, putting bowls of food on the table, and allowing everyone to serve themselves. This not only decreases the temptation to make kids eat what's on their plate, it helps children get used to taking how much food they think they are hungry for, knowing they can go back for more if they want.

When you consistently offer food and allow kids to decide how much to eat, you will be amazed at how well they can regulate their food intake. One study found that middle-school children who scored high on intuitive eating had lower BMIs, less body dissatisfaction and pressure to be thin, and were more likely to be satisfied with life.[6]

Sitting down to meals also helps kids attentively eat. Emerging research shows paying attention is a powerful ally in appetite control, not just at meals but also for how much is eaten later in the day.

The Power of Paying Attention

As a young child, I remember sitting down to family dinners, but as I got older this stopped. We had those cool TV tray tables that allowed us to eat while watching TV (for those of you who grew up in the 1970s you can probably relate). As I grew into an adult and still wasn't paying attention at meals, I didn't even know this was a problem. Like many things in our culture, it just became a normal behavior. I was hungry all the time, but it never dawned on me that sitting down and paying attention was the antidote. That was, until my dietetic internship where I had to go to the hospital for main meals and had nowhere to keep food in my dorm. Once I discovered the benefits of focusing on meals, I never went back to my previous mindless eating.

In one study of eating habits, researchers separated female college students into three groups. At a lunch meal, one group focused on the sensory qualities of the food, the second read an article while eating, and the third just ate as normal. Later when offered cookies, the first group who paid close attention to what they were eating not only ate less cookies but rated their appetite as lower than the other two groups.[7]

The reason for this is what researchers call "episodic meal memory." When we pay attention at meals, we remember that meal more and eat less the next time. Research suggests that eating while distracted affects intake at the immediate meal somewhat, but has an even greater effect on later eating. In short, being distracted while eating lunch could mean eating more than you need at dinner.[8]

There are many real-life examples of this. You read a few pages of a book but aren't paying attention so you have to reread those pages next time. You are on the phone while checking email and are asked a question you have no idea how to answer. Or my worst one, not paying attention to what my husband said in the morning and calling him later to ask for the bit of information he imparted to me (busted!).

It's a fairly simple concept. When we fail to pay attention while we eat, the meal doesn't register in our brain the way it should. So when we go to eat later, we forget about what we ate and are likely to eat more than our bodies need.

Can Food Regulation Skills Be Taught?

Thirty children were tested on their ability to regulate food intake. The researchers found that some regulated their food intake well, others over-ate, and a third group under-ate. Then the children went through a six-week program where they were taught how the stomach gets full using dolls. After the program, those that over-ate and those that under-ate showed better food regulation. Some kids even said things like "I can't have more soup, I'm too full."[9]

This begs the question…if children aren't regulating their food intake now, can they be taught? While this study hints to the answer being yes, we need more research. I believe parents and caregivers can certainly help kids "tune in" to their internal signals of eating. While changing feeding practices is more important, some kids may need additional help identifying internal signals.

One key way to do this is to incorporate language that helps kids become aware of what is going on with their bodies. When observed, child-care providers at Head Start failed to give hunger and fullness cues when asking children if they want to eat more – for example, asking children if they want more food without referring to being full, telling children to eat, and using praise to encourage children to eat more.[10]

Researchers call helping children recognize hunger and fullness "intake coaching." This is when parents accept their children's hunger cues and help to guide these children to appropriate choices. For example, this could be helping children assess how hungry they are before taking food, asking children if they're full or have more room for more when offering food, and reminding children when the next eating occasion is so they can effectively manage their hunger.

Intake Coaching	
Instead of...	**Say...**
• Are you done? • Want more? • I think you had enough (in response to asking for more food) • Please take X more bites	• Are you full or still hungry? • What does your tummy say? Is it full or hungry for more? • Make sure you filled your belly; we won't be eating until dinnertime

Another important way to drive these points home is to make it part of your family food culture. "Our culture [around food] becomes pretty invisible and normal," said Megrette Fletcher M.Ed., R.D., CDE, author of *Discover*

Mindful Eating for Kids. It pays to be intentional about the food culture you create in your home. In her book, Fletcher has a list of mindful-eating principles that you can choose from, to help you describe your desired food culture. She shares an example of how she created a culture with her family around "Becoming Aware of Physical Hunger":

> *In my home, as soon as my children were old enough (about 3-4 years old), they began to serve themselves. In the 10 years since I started doing this, it has become a 'house' rule. Friends, family and dinner guests are informed that this is how we serve food. There is a pause before service where everyone does a 'tummy check' and then chooses an amount of food to meet this hunger level. In the beginning this step was more formal; by now – it is quick, often invisible when we are not entertaining. However, when there is an audience, a tummy check can become an opportunity for my children to break into a song and dance routine (kids can be creative, fun and crazy, which is why I love them!).*[11]

The key is to make paying attention at meals and listening to internal cues the norm, or what Fletcher calls an "invisible habit." Your kids will thank you when they are adults.

The Child Who Never Seems Full

Occasionally, I hear from a parent that believes her child doesn't register fullness. This type of situation causes a lot of stress for families. Some kids sneak food and may even throw up if allowed to eat as much as they want. There are some medical conditions, like Prader Willi, that can cause eating problems, but these are not common. Sometimes medications and behavioral issues can cause an over- or underactive appetite. I always recommend parents get a medical checkup to reassure them nothing is physically causing this eating problem. Oftentimes, these families need professional help to turn things around. I highly suggest finding someone with a feeding dynamics background, who will consider not just what a child is being fed but also the how and why of feeding (recommendations at the end of the book).

The literature shows, though, that some kids have more trouble controlling their food impulses for a variety of nonmedical reasons. Sometimes temperament is a problem, and the parent may have used food to help soothe their difficult child, especially when they were a baby. For example, children rated as highly emotional were twice as likely to be overweight approaching age ten, compared to other children not rated this way.[12]

I suspect problems of this magnitude often begin when the child is young. Like Marci's story, it might be that the baby was restricted early in life or that an always-crying baby was fed more due to a very difficult temperament. In one study, 279 first-time mothers of babies taught responsive parenting, which focused on feeding, sleep, and emotional regulation, were less likely to have overweight children by age one than those not taught these strategies.[13] "Feeding a baby can be an easy and fast way to quiet an upset baby," said Jennifer Savage, assistant professor of nutritional sciences at Penn State. "But we don't want parents to use feeding to soothe their baby if the baby isn't hungry – crying is one of the last things a baby is likely to do if they are hungry. By getting to know their baby's temperament and establishing predictable routines early in life, parents are able to help their baby learn self-regulation."[14]

Sometimes problems don't happen until a bit later. From my interactions with parents, I find eating problems tend to occur around the age of three. This is a time when children become more aware of their environment and may start asking for more sweets. They also become more picky at this time, another frustration for parents. A child who feels deprived may start to zero in on goodie foods and engage in the cycle of eating when not hungry. The next principle details what to do in these cases.

One way of looking at eating challenges is that some children simply need more support than others. Certain children are harder to feed and it's not the kids' or parents' fault. The 8 Principles in this book are designed to get at all the possible reasons a child is having trouble regulating their food intake. If you find that allowing kids to eat until they are full is not working, Principles 7 and 8 should be particularly helpful.

Allow Hunger and Fullness to Guide Eating Summary

Allowing internal cues to guide eating is simple in theory, but may be one of the most difficult things a parent can do. There are times your child will eat the way you want them to eat and other times they won't. If you've been controlling how much they eat, you can expect that they initially will make mistakes. This doesn't mean it's not working but rather that your child is learning how to manage their own hunger, and as with anything, mistakes teach lessons. If they are used to being stopped during eating, they may overeat for a while with the newfound freedom, but this should eventually wane.

Here are the main tips from Principle 2 about allowing hunger and fullness to guide eating:

1) Avoid distractions, like the TV or devices, at eating time. Have a designated place to eat and make your eating space visually appealing when possible.

2) Be mindful of the wonderful taste and texture of the food that's being eaten. Leave judgment out of eating (yours and your kid's), which is a surefire way to stir up distraction.

3) Provide verbal cues about what was eaten before to refresh your memory. I believe this is easier when you have a structured eating style, but I often remind my kids of what they ate, especially when saying no to requests for certain items ("Remember, we already had chips, ice cream, etc.").

4) Serve meals family style, placing food in bowls on the table, and encourage kids to take as much as they think they will be hungry for. Less is better as they can always have more, as we try not to waste food.

5) Although you can guide your child to increase their awareness of hunger and fullness, it is ultimately up to each child to decide how much to eat. Refer to internal cues when offering more food ("Are you full or are you still hungry for more?").

You will be relieved as you see your son or daughter get enough food to eat. You no longer are doing a job for which you were never qualified to do, so that struggle will disappear. Everybody knows what their body needs, if they can learn to just listen.

Next, we focus on how to handle those palatable foods kids are naturally drawn to.

PRINCIPLE 3

NEUTRALIZE THE POWER OF GOODIES

"If you don't love it, don't eat it, and if you love it, savor it."–Evelyn Tribole

There's a cultural phenomenon showing that negative attention draws intense interest. Remember the negative reviews Miley Cyrus got for her performance at the VMAs in 2013? Her record sales skyrocketed at that time. And after every one of those horrible shootings, the media gives the killers so much press time that internet searches for them go through the roof.

Sweets, fried food, and starchy snacks – what I call "goodies"– all get this same kind of treatment. We hype them up, make them bad, tightly control them, or worse yet, have them around all the time and then use them as a reward for good behavior. Goodies are what they are, something to enjoy at certain times. The more attention we give to them, the more fixated on goodies children become.

Because kids are naturally drawn to goodies, the key is to neutralize their potential for power.

This principle is for children over two only. That's because during the first two years there is no need to regularly offer children sweets or empty-calorie foods. Their stomachs are small and their nutrition needs high. Plus, they are not even aware of these foods in the first place. That being said, having a little here and there is fine, but as for regular offerings wait until your child is two, and starts to show interest.

The goal for this third principle is to teach children how to include goodies into a balanced diet without all the typical baggage that makes them even more desirable.

The Food Framework – Remove, Reward, Repeat

Carla was constantly on her three kids about eating goodies, telling them to eat small portions or to eat healthy before anything sweet. She thought limiting how much children eat is how you teach moderation. On the flip side, she also used sweets to get her kids to behave, do chores, and finish their homework. She tried other rewards but nothing worked like candy. She often threatened to take dessert away if they behaved badly, and that always got them to straighten up.

You could say this strategy worked. Her kids stopped eating when she told them to, and they ate real food before having dessert. But there were also signs it wasn't working, like discovering one of her kids raided his friend's fridge or traded his healthy lunch. When Carla couldn't be there to control her children's eating, there was trouble.

Bubbling below the surface was her kids' growing desire for sweets. With each nag, reward, and punishment that included food, she was giving goodies more power. Her children already knew these items tasted good, but with all the fanfare, they were taking on even more meaning. They also were learning that they couldn't trust themselves around sweets, as their mom made it clear that they needed tight control.

Turn Up the Focus

You know what it's like when you discover something new and then see it everywhere. You buy a blue car for the first time, and suddenly everyone seems to have a blue car. You go through a certain experience, like a car accident, and find that many others have had that same experience. The world hasn't changed but your focus has. In short, the mind fixates on what we choose to focus on, even when it's something we aren't supposed to do. When Carla nagged her kids about goodies, this only turned up the focus on these foods, so they ate more when they had the chance. The reason for this is what researchers call 'ironic processes' as described in the Position Paper for European Childhood Obesity Group:

'Control', with its necessity to maintain 'restrained eating' at the meta-level, describes how the human brain is principally unable not to think about something. Every 'control' thought, like 'I am not going to eat chocolate and chips now' activates an image of chocolate, etc., in the brain, similar to a search command on a computer for 'NOT obesity' which will open all files and text passages containing the word 'obesity'. Consequently, the suppressed thoughts become even more conscious through so-called 'ironic processes' that overload the individual's mental processes, and thus paradoxically, the unwanted behaviour (e.g., eating more of a favourite snack having abstained from

it for 24 h). [1]

Rewarding and punishing children with food also turns up the food focus. In one study, parents of eight- to twelve-year-olds were asked about their child's daily food intake and whether they used what researchers call "control food rules." The parents who used food to control behavior had kids who ate significantly more calories, carbohydrates, and fat. [2] Adults who recall their parents using food to control behavior through reward and punishment were more likely to use dietary restraint (restricting food practices such as dieting) and binge-eat. [3]

Where did these ideas about feeding start? Research suggests parental concern for a child's weight is often an instigator. In the controversial book *The Heavy*, Dara-Lynn Weiss shares how her concern for her child's weight resulted in restrictive dieting to lose weight. [4] Yet many of the food issues seemed to be about the mom, not the child. Research shows this connection between a mom's and child's eating is real. For instance, when moms score high on levels of intuitive eating, they are less likely to use restriction even when concerned about their child's weight. But when mothers score low or average on intuitive eating, they are more likely to use restriction with their kids. [5] Additionally, when a mother feels out of control eating certain foods or eats to manage difficult emotions, her child is more likely to do the same. [6,7]

There can be a significant mismatch between the lens through which a parent and a child see food. A child overeats cookies because he hasn't had them in a while, for instance, but the parent assumes it's because he has no self-control. After a while — and with certain feeding practices — the child can adopt the parent's outlook on food. So it's worth it to take the time to see if there are any connections between your relationship with food, your feeding style, and your child's eating.

Why Children Crave Carbs

Children are motivated by satisfying eating experiences and are biologically driven to prefer sweet tastes. Starting in infancy with breast milk, sweet tastes signify a safe source of energy, while bitter can signal danger.[8] That being said, most infants eat a large variety of food but tend to narrow down this variety around age two.

As children reach toddlerhood, growth declines in terms of the body but increases when it comes to metabolic needs of the brain. Researchers from Northwestern University discovered that glucose uptake peaks during the slow period of growth between toddlerhood and puberty in order for the brain to fully develop. The brain relies heavily on glucose, which is why a child's brain uses up twice as much glucose as an adult brain does. Brain glucose requirements peak at about five years of age (almost half of daily energy intake goes to the brain!), years before adult brain size is reached.[9] This may be why young kids tend to go for the starchy foods first and why preference for sweets tends to increase after the baby and young toddler phase.

Carb-rich foods continue to play a key role as children grow and develop. When children and young adults were separated by age and given a taste test, the school age children (9-10) preferred the higher sweet concentrations more than the adolescents (14-16). The adolescents preferred higher sweet intensities than the adults (20-25).[10] One study took things a step further and children were categorized into high- and low-sweet preferences. These two groups did not differ by age, body weight, stage of puberty, height, or gender. Where they did differ is a measurement referred to as NTx, a marker of bone growth that can be detected in urine. The results showed that the children that were still growing showed a heightened preference for sweets compared to those who had stopped growing (around 15-16).[11] "I don't know for sure, but I am very suspicious that the bones are somehow telling either the brain or the tongue that there is energy needed for their growth and signaling for that preference to increase," said lead researcher Nancy Coldwell in an interview on NPR.[12] The following point is also made in the published study:

This elegant link between taste preferences and biological need may leave modern children especially vulnerable to the long-term consequences of overeating and caries in the advent of an abundant sugar supply. However if we accept sugar liking as a natural concomitant to growth in childhood, then it brings into question the assumption that this propensity is invariably unhealthy and undesirable among this age group.

Children may be more vulnerable due to their taste preferences, but these taste preferences also play a role in growth. In short, you don't need to sweat the fact that your child loves carbs, and it's pretty normal for her to eat more than you do. But it's also important to handle goodies with special care, which is what the rest of this principle focuses on.

Let's see how a Mindful Framework helps you give the power to your child, instead of food.

The Mindful Framework – Enjoy, Plan and Stop Rewarding

When Carla changed her approach to a mindful one, she was able to see that her attempts at controlling her kids' sweet intake – and behavior with food – wasn't working. In reality, her kids never seemed motivated to do their homework or help around the house of their own volition. Also, they didn't eat small portions of sweets when she wasn't around. Using food in this way did not appear to be a long-term solution. She also realized that she never learned how to eat goodies in moderation either. She suspected her own distrust around sweets may be part of the reason she was so hard on her kids.

Although it seemed counterintuitive, she gave her children permission to enjoy goodies. In other words, they got to eat nag-free within the structure of mealtime and snacks. When she offered goodies as a snack, they were able to eat until they were satisfied. Other times, like with dinner or closer to bed, smaller portions were called for. When she said no to sweet requests outside of this structure, she explained why in a calm and empathetic way. She stopped using food to reward and punish her children. Instead, she set up a routine where they needed to do chores and homework before screen time.

Because her kids were no longer being nagged and offered goodies for other reasons, they stopped fixating on them. Her children learned how these foods fit into a balanced diet. Slowly but surely, they developed perceived control over goodies. Carla was so inspired, she started to make some changes herself.

Won't My Child Go Crazy?

Researchers separated children into three groups. One group of children were forbidden to eat sweets, the other was forbidden from eating fruit, and the third group was told they could eat as much as they wanted of all the food. When the food was made freely available to all three groups, the unrestricted kids consumed the least. Not only that, they reported less desire for sweets compared to the other two (restricted) groups.[13]

Giving children wiggle room around goodies is justified for important reasons. First, when kids know they can have as much as they want of something, it decreases in power. Think about it. Marketers don't tell you the sale is *always* available. They use scarcity to get people to act, letting them know the sale won't be offered after a certain date. Without this type of shortage, people don't feel compelled to do anything. Same goes with food — when it's not scarce, the need to act is diminished.

Eating with pleasure – instead of guilt – also has benefits. In one study, people who associated eating chocolate with guilt versus celebration, were more likely to report unhealthy eating habits, perceived themselves as unhealthy eaters when stressed, and used food for mood regulation.[14] When we eat for pleasure it's allowed, but when there's guilt it feels naughty and people often need excuses to eat (like stress or bad feelings), which leads to overeating.

None of this means we should line our cabinets with goodies and eat them nonstop. The amount of exposure we give our children certainly matters.

The Exposure Effect

A survey with 670 college students and their parents revealed something most research agrees with: Frequent food exposure matters in the development of long-term food preferences. The nutritious and not-so-nutritious foods the young adults preferred were strongly related to the foods they saw repeatedly in childhood. This was even true for items they disliked as kids.[15]

Just because restriction can increase a child's focus on certain foods doesn't mean they benefit from a steady supply of goodies. In fact, it's up to you which foods you surround your child with. In the study, the foods kids weren't exposed to in childhood were more likely to be disliked in young adulthood.

This has to do with covert versus overt control. Parents utilize covert control simply by limiting what foods come into the house, choosing quality food products, and deciding how often different items show up in the structure of feeding. So maybe dessert is skipped when a child had something sweet already or chips aren't served with dinner to balance the meal out. Monitoring a child's eating and serving food accordingly makes sense. This is different from overt control such as nagging a kid each time they reach in the cookie jar, always limiting their portion of sweets, or leaving tasty food in sight and saying no repeatedly.

- *Covert control:* taking charge of what food is in the home and how it is served
- *Overt control:* controlling the child instead of the environment

So put some thought into the foods you have in your house – goodies and otherwise – and ask yourself if you are exposing your kids to the type of variety you want them to eat if not now, then someday. The foods they are exposed to the most frequently will be the ones they will prefer when they are out on their own.

How a Flexible Goodies Policy Can Help

Providing a regular and consistent offering of goodies is what I call a flexible goodies policy (FGP). When the right offerings occur, children are calm around sweets. They still love them and may eat quite a bit at times, but they understand their role in the diet and that they will get them again. There's no need to sneak, hide, or feel guilty for eating something so enjoyable.

There are two aspects to your goodies policy to consider: *How often* and *how much*. Unfortunately, research can't tell us the best course of action for every family. *How often* will depend on your preferences as a family. International feeding expert Ellyn Satter recommends serving a small portion of dessert with dinner to level the playing field with other foods. The key is not to allow seconds and give children the freedom to eat the food in any order they want.[16] Jill Castle, pediatric nutrition expert, recommends a 90:10 rule for older kids. "For most healthy kids, a good rule of thumb is to eat no more than one-to-two Fun Foods each day," she said. "Kids can understand this concept — and the best part – allowing kids to choose which Fun Food they will eat."[17]

Marci, from the introduction, said she made tweaks along the way to her FGP based on what was and wasn't working. For example, she tried to keep it to one treat a day but then she found her daughter would lie about having sweets outside the home, like a lollipop, so she let it go. She even stopped asking what her children ate outside the home. "The less I mention the sweets, the better they regulate," she said.

After a blog post on the subject, one of my readers decided to end the dinnertime negotiations with her children (ages six and eight) by asking for their input. "What we came up with is that they can have dessert two nights a week whether or not they eat much dinner or how many veggies they eat." When I checked in with her a year later, she said the treat solution was still working, with an extra weeknight dessert added for special occasions. "The treat night solution has cut out a great deal of dinner frustration for me since it eliminates the question *did I eat enough to get a treat?"* she said. Her kids do question it every once in a while but she is quick to point out how many outside treats they get throughout the week at school, church, and other places.

The *how much* is a little trickier. I personally believe it's important to have times kids are allowed to eat goodies until they are satisfied as long as they pay attention and stay at the table. In addition to dessert with dinner, Satter recommends offering goodies once a week allowing kids to eat as much as they want. This freedom around sweets may be especially important for the child who is acting out due to previous restriction. "We have noticed big changes even in just one month," said Andrea, explaining how her preschooler's interest in candy decreased after about ten days without restriction. "The control over her food (specifically sugar) had become quite a stress in our lives and changing our ways was also a challenge."

In our family, we have a flexible once-a-day policy. We typically enjoy sweets like dark chocolate, baked goods, and ice cream daily, although on weekends it can be more and other days none. At parties and snack time, kids are free to eat as much as they want as long as they stay at the table. When dessert is after dinner, sometimes the amount is limited if it's close to bedtime. Now that my kids are getting older (seven and ten), more often than not, they stop on their own. Some families may opt to offer sweets less often, and this can work out fine, too. Table P3.1 provides a summary of FGP options and considerations.

Your flexible goodies policy will be personal and something you feel is right for your family. Just be willing to change it if you sense it's not working or if your child is fixating on food.

Table P3.1 FGP Options		
Flexible Goodies Policy	*What is it?*	*Potential Watch-outs*
Satter's Dessert with Dinner	Serve a small portion of dessert with dinner allowing kids to eat in any order. Have another time (like afternoon snack) during the week kids can eat sweets until satisfaction.	Might be hard for older kids to make this transition. Also, parents may start to feel obligated to always have dessert with dinner.
Castle's 90:10 Rule	Allow kids to choose their own one-two goodies per day. Amount: a typical serving size.	Some kids may feel restricted if unable to eat until satisfaction. This tends to work better for older children who understand 90:10 concept.
Flexible Once a Day	Unspoken rule of one sweet per day. Exceptions made for parties and weekends with lots of activities. Amount eaten typically left up to children, although limits can be made under certain circumstances.	Some kids may do better on fewer sweets or need more structure and guidance.
Occasional Sweets	Keeping sweets to occasional 1-2 times per week or weekends only.	Some kids may feel deprived with occasional treats, and start to fixate on such foods.

- *Signs it's working:* Children asking or whining for sweets at times is normal. Overall, you feel your child is satisfied with how often they get goodies and they don't overly fixate on them. They may eat a lot of something they haven't had in a while, but when they are done they stop thinking about it.
- *Signs it's not working:* A child that is constantly asking for sweets and never seems satisfied after eating them. He may even start sneaking or you see that he consistently goes crazy with sweets outside of the home. When this happens, it's time to change things.

Problem Solving

I find parents typically have lots of questions about different situations involving goodies. Here are some potential scenarios, contributing factors, and language to help you find resolution.

Takes a bite or two of dinner, then devours dessert

It just doesn't feel right to have a kid who barely touches dinner but eats dessert with gusto. Here are some potential causes to address:

- Was there something at the dinner table the child liked? I always suggest parents provide at least one if not two items kids accept at mealtime. If there are too many unfamiliar foods at dinner, kids may hold out for dessert.
- Is dessert always after dinner? Try to not make this the habit kids expect. Try sweets earlier in the day or if your child is a toddler that doesn't eat well at dinner, which is typical, try serving a more wholesome dessert-

- or try Satter's dessert with dinner to help get you through this not-into-dinner stage.

- Be sure that for at least two hours before dinner there's no snacking so kids can build up an appetite.

Keeps asking if they had enough to eat to earn dessert

Kids used to eating to earn dessert may keep asking you if they ate enough. Be sure they understand that what or how much they eat at dinner is not tied to dessert: "The food at dinner should fill you up, dessert is just to fill that sweet craving. You don't have to eat a certain amount of anything to get dessert!"

Never seems satisfied

You created your flexible goodies policy and your child still doesn't seem satisfied and continues to fixate on sweet treats.

- If you just started your FGP, be patient and give it time to see if it works. If after a while you still notice your kid's fixation, try increasing offerings if you are occasional or cutting back if it's once a day. Also, be sure your child is aware of the FGP so he knows what to expect.

- Some pickier kids may flock to energy-dense foods because they fill them up easily. Be sure they have enough food to fill them up at meals and snacks. Bring your child into the process: "How do you feel about meals and snacks? Are you satisfied or is there something you'd like to see?"

- If nothing you do seems to help, check Principles 6, 7, and 8 to see if a fixation on goodies is due to stress, lack of self-care like sleep and exercise, or dealing with difficult feelings and circumstances.

Teaching Lessons

Along with structure, a flexible goodies policy and using covert control, teaching kids the following lessons makes a difference.

Put stuff out of sight

The researchers I've talked with all agree that the most damaging thing to kids is to have food right in front of them but saying they cannot have it. "Having food in sight but off limits drives kids crazy," said Jennifer Orlet Fisher, PhD, Associate Professor in the Department of Public Health at Temple University. "Caregivers need to decide what's appropriate to bring in the house and how accessible they want to make it."

This isn't a keep-it-out-of-the-house type of advice, but simply having a designated place for goodies, taking items out when it's time to eat, and then putting them away.

Find non-food ways to soothe

When kids experience difficult feelings, it's easy to offer the cookie for the scraped knee or the lollipop following shots at the doctor. While once in a while this is fine, too much of this can create an association that sweets are needed to make bad feelings go away.

Although kids benefit from getting their feelings out (see Principle 8 for more), you can work with them on non-food ways to help themselves feel better. Maybe they like to listen to music or get outside to play or take a warm bath or even call a family member. Doing something that feels good – and feeds the spirit – helps your child see problems and difficult feelings in a new light.

Parties and natural consequences

You can feel like you do everything right at home, but then get to parties or to the grandparents' home, and it becomes a free-for-all with food. I struggled with this early on but decided that allowing my children, especially when young, freedom to choose was good for a few reasons. First, it was interesting to see what they chose on their own. Second, they could experience natural consequences if they ate too much or too little.

Instead of an "I told you so" if a child isn't feeling so hot due to poor choices at a party, help them discover the source. Once they realize it was the food, you can remind them the next time so they make the connection sooner.

Be picky

You hear a lot about the perils of picky eating in childhood, but when it comes to goodies, being picky is the lesson you *want* to teach. You can up the ante by providing homemade desserts, wholesome treats, and dark chocolate at home instead of packaged treats that are lower in quality (and in my opinion, taste). The idea is for kids to learn to appreciate – and even become picky about the kind of sweets they enjoy.

Halloween is actually a good time to teach children about being a selective candy eater. Have children sort through their stash and pick their favorite items, giving the mediocre ones away. Of course, they can try the items they've never had before deciding if they're worth keeping.

The first few bites are the best

Explain to your kids about how food enjoyment declines as a food is being eaten — something researchers call "sensory-specific satiety." In other words, the first few bites of eating are the most enjoyable. This is particularly important for eating sweets, a food that's meant for pleasure not nourishment.

The key is to teach kids to be mindful, that enjoyment comes early in the eating experience, and frequent eating of indulgent foods makes them less enjoyable. So if it's a day when sweets will be offered multiple times, encourage them to choose the one they think they will enjoy the most. Over time, children learn to be selective and that they really don't need that much of the sweet stuff, when they do eat it.

<u>Neutralize the Power of Goodies Summary</u>

There's a lot to digest and work on in this principle. Just as Rome wasn't built in a day, managing goodies takes time. Here are Principle 3's key points:

1) Consider your own relationship with food, and how that affects the way you feed your child.
2) Remember children prefer sweet foods more so than adults, and this is at least partially biologically driven. In other words, nothing's wrong when they enjoy and even whine for sweets.

3) Be neutral about goodies and avoid giving them added attention. That means not using sweets to reward, punish, or soothe uncomfortable feelings. No need to lecture kids on how "bad" they are for health either.

4) Create and be consistent with a flexible goodies policy, your rhythm of sweet offerings during the week. Send the message that sweets are an enjoyable part of the diet and not something to feel guilty about.

5) To avoid scarcity, have times where kids can eat goodies until satisfied – such as during one or two snack times a week – as long as they stay at the table while eating. For example, homemade cookies with milk for their afternoon snack.

6) Teach lessons throughout kids' lives such as being selective, savoring sweets, and having a designated place for goodies in the house.

Now that we put goodies in their place, you'll want to give your attention to the nourishing foods you want your kids to eat.

PRINCIPLE 4

MAKE NUTRITION A
REWARDING PART OF EATING

"In my food world there is no fear or guilt, only joy and abundance." –Ellie Krieger

Researchers at the University of Chicago sought to find out how healthy-eating information affects children's eating. One of three groups of preschool children was read a story about how crackers made a girl big and strong, giving her lots of energy. The second group was read a story about how the crackers tasted good, making the girl happy. The third group of children was not read a story. Later, when the kids were given fifteen crackers to eat, children in the healthy group ate the least (three) compared to those in the yummy (seven), and the no story group (nine). Another experiment using carrots showed similar results.[1]

This phenomenon is alive and well in our current environment. At a time where nutrition information is seemingly growing on trees, it still hasn't spurred people into long-term action. And in some cases, as this study shows, it can have the opposite effect.

Research suggests that as children get older they increasingly view healthy food as inferior in the taste department.[2] This has real implications as children – who turn into adults – seek satisfying eating experiences. The key is to raise children with a healthy mindset, meaning they view nutritious foods in a positive and satisfying light. This is vital for raising a mindful eater, and this chapter will show you how.

The Food Framework – Define Healthy and Unhealthy

Tim was a nutrition enthusiast and wanted his kids to eat healthy like he does. He often pointed out which foods were "healthy" and "unhealthy." His kids loved this on a conceptual level because they are concrete thinkers, and they often asked: Is this healthy? Is that healthy? In the process of gathering evidence about food, they began to view healthy food as a separate entity from regular and tasty eating. Tim didn't understand how they could recite which foods were healthy but still didn't choose these foods on their own. In fact, as they got older they seemed to resent this nutrition talk and became even more defiant.

Although health was important to Tim, it wasn't (yet) to his children. Like most kids, they were interested in satisfying eating experiences, not their long-term health. So when it came time to eat, they picked foods they thought would be most satisfying. They began to look at "healthy" food as an obligation, as their dad also required they eat a certain amount at each meal. The more disinterested in healthy eating his children seemed, the stronger Tim's resolve to teach them became, and he created even more rules around eating.

Tim's kids were developing a conflicting relationship with food since they knew their dad wanted them to eat healthy but they associated such foods with inferior taste. And even though they knew they shouldn't enjoy unhealthy foods, they associated them with the most pleasure.

Why Nutrition Knowledge Doesn't Translate to Behavior

Most people assume that educating children about nutrition is the key to good eating. The research does not necessarily back this up. In a group of seven- to thirteen-year-olds, those under eleven with the most nutrition knowledge consumed less unhealthy foods. But the children over eleven, with the most nutrition knowledge, did not consume less unhealthy foods.[3] In this age group, taste and social acceptability were the only factors related to consumption. One study that performed focus groups with children came to this conclusion:

Healthy foods appeared to be conceptualized largely in terms of food groups and nutrients, whereas liked and unhealthy foods were conceptualized in relation to taste, texture, and visual appeal... Across all ages, taste factored more into descriptions of liked and unhealthy foods.[4]

This can lead to something researchers call expected satiety. If healthy items are thought of as less satisfying, they may leave people dissatisfied. Take a study where adults were given the same energy bar but one was presented as "tasty" and the other as "healthy." After eating the bar, the healthy group reported higher levels of hunger than the tasty group.[5]

Researchers of the aforementioned cracker study

speculate that when kids are told food serves one goal (health), they may view it as less tied to another goal (taste). This can even happen when children already like something healthy. Research shows that being rewarded and praised for doing something you already enjoy, can decrease motivation for it.[6] So if Pam starts being praised for eating broccoli, something she willingly eats, she may start to question if she's eating it for the praise or because she really likes it.

This doesn't mean nutrition should never be mentioned, it just means we need to be mindful about the real effect it's having.

Nutrition Education with a Negative Slant

Another common way to educate kids about nutrition is to focus on the negative consequences that can happen by eating certain foods. "Don't eat this because it's bad for you" is often used. Sometimes long-term consequences are mentioned like a family history of diabetes or heart disease.

Focusing on the negative consequences in terms of health advice is not only ineffective at creating change, it can increase pleasure from the forbidden item. In one study, people primed with guilt like getting reminders about their health and looking at fitness magazines, reported more enjoyment from sweets. This study found an association between guilt and pleasure that most of the people in the study were not aware of.[7]

This may happen more with kids because preference for sweet and energy-rich food is universal and driven by growth and development. Even in countries like France where families share traditional meals, kids' favorite foods still include items like fried potatoes, chocolate cake, and sweet nut spread.[8] When kids are constantly told the foods they are slow to warm up to (like vegetables) are good for them, and the foods they love are bad for them, it can solidify early in life that bad foods equal pleasure.

So if this way of educating kids can backfire, what's a more effective way to build the attitudes and actions you want? Keep it positive, meaningful, and satisfying!

The Mindful Framework – Making Nutrition a Want-to

With a Mindful Framework, Tim did some digging first. He thought about how he got interested in nutrition in the first place, realizing this didn't happen until he got into cross-country running as a teenager. Before that he mostly cared how food tasted and satisfied him. There was no one trying to get him to eat healthy, and he did eat nutritious food but just because it was part of the food his parents had around. He could see that it wasn't until he was internally motivated towards nutritious eating, that he began to make healthy choices. He realized all the nagging and food rules were having the opposite effect on his kids.

So Tim stopped the food rules at the table and nagging his children to choose healthy foods. When he could, he helped them make the connection between food and positive effects, especially things they found meaningful. For example, for his son he'd say "You have basketball practice later, so let's eat something that will give you lasting energy." Or with his daughter who loved sweets, he'd remind her before a party how she felt last time she ate too much cake. He also focused on finding tasty ways to prepare wholesome food and enjoying it himself without announcing how healthy it was. Tim made a point to bring his kids into the cooking process, which piqued their curiosity for food in general.

Slowly but surely, his kids began to associate healthy food with taste and satisfaction. They also started to make the connection between the food they ate, and how they felt physically. Although they didn't always make the healthy choice, Tim noticed how they freely chose nutritious foods at least some of the time (without him hammering them!), and he knew this desire would grow as they got older.

Nutrition Information – The Positive Spin

Three-to seven-year-olds were read stories such as "Pinocchio," "The Boy Who Cried Wolf," and "George Washington and the Cherry Tree." The latter story, which focuses on the positive effects of telling the truth, increased truth telling in the children, while the other stories that focused on the negative consequences of not telling the truth, didn't.[9]

In the same way, focusing on how eating well positively effects one's life is more motivating than making the choice to avoid bad outcomes. In one study, family and home experiences with food like gardening together helped shape positive attitudes and likeability of nutritious foods. As one girl said, "We have a garden at our house, and we grow corn, cucumbers, and potatoes," and that she liked "...to eat foods from the garden."[10] Good teachers know that desire and interest are key to helping children learn. In particular, active engagement, curiosity, joy, learning from mistakes, and continued effort is key.[11]

Even the way health professionals like dietitians counsel people is changing. 'Out' are the days of just telling people what to do, and 'in' is a popular communication tool called motivational interviewing. It's a counseling method focused on helping individuals become intrinsically motivated to make healthy changes, and it's been shown to be effective with children.[12] It's all about the client coming up with solutions and figuring out for themselves where the true barriers and benefits lie. One key aspect of motivational interviewing to keep in mind is supporting and encouraging children to explore – and find meaningful – the benefits of healthy habits for themselves. This is much better than always rushing to give them the answer.

Some ways to support children include pointing out the roles different foods play, instead of labeling items as "good" or "bad." You can help children see that some foods do a better job of nourishing the body than other foods do – which is why we eat some foods more or less often – but no one food can do it all. It's the combination of a variety of food that increases satisfaction and makes people healthy and children grow. Also, allowing kids to learn from mistakes with natural consequences from eating "out of balance" is much more powerful than always telling them that something is harmful or bad.

When we raise kids with a positive and balanced approach to eating well, they don't feel conflicted about their natural inclinations towards food. They grow up seeing balanced eating and moving their body as a regular and rewarding part of their life, not some obligation they need to fulfill. But of course there's more – getting kids involved in the process.

Nutrition Education for Kids: What we Know

There is no shortage of attempts to educate kids about nutrition both in schools and at home. Schools often have programs or health classes for kids. According to one review, experiential or hands-on learning produced the best outcomes such as increased knowledge and a preference for fruits and vegetables. Yet they are the least likely to be used in class in favor of curriculum-based learning.[13,14]

Curriculum-based learning makes sense for teaching reading, writing, and math. For kids to become good readers, they need to learn to sound out words and put them together to form sentences before they can read stories. Same with writing and math, learn a small bit at a time, practice, and move on. Food is actually the opposite. Because children don't have the ability to think abstractly about nutrition until they are older, messages like "fruit is high in vitamin C" or "we eat foods without artificial additives" aren't effective. Worse yet, when they are given too many details too early, kids' concrete minds turn the information into absolutes.[15] What children really need is more exposure and experience with different foods before they can apply the nutrition part.

Take a pilot study done with nine-year-olds. One-third of the class was given educational materials about the benefits of eating fruit, another third weren't given anything at all (the control group), and the last third was exposed to fruit by their teacher. At the end of the intervention, the education and exposure groups increased their fruit intake. But it was only the exposure group that kept eating fruit a year later. We also know that children who regularly cook eat more fruits and vegetables than those who don't.[16] In the early years, it makes sense to focus on the experiential learning for kids while providing teachable moments. As they get older, they will ask nutrition questions, which I believe is the best way to learn because the interest is there. With a solid foundation about food, how it's prepared and pulled together for balance, nutrition information presented later can be the icing on the cake. After all, kids in high school benefit from knowing how to read a label, interpret advertising, and a whole slew of other nutrition topics.

Nutrition education is not what makes kids eat and prefer a variety of food. It's the daily exposure and learning about food that gets them involved. Yet nutrition education at the right time, with a solid foundation of different food experiences and preferences, adds great value.

A Bit About the WHAT

In the last principle, I mention a study about food exposure to goodies and its effect on eating in young adulthood. That same study showed that the college students ate the same healthy foods they were exposed to as kids, even when they didn't prefer them early in life. Children learn by example both by what is offered and what their parents eat. Even though it may take years for them to get around to eating salad, seeing it weekly at the kitchen table is slowly working its magic. In fact, the foods you choose to frequently expose your children to is very powerful.

What you serve your kids also matters in terms of nutrition, hunger, and satiety. Balanced meals and snacks are more satisfying and filling than single foods. What's going to be more satisfying? A bunch of crackers or crackers with cheese and fruit? A good rule of thumb is to provide two-to-three food groups for snack and three-to-five at main meals. Food groups include grains/starchy food, fruits, vegetables, protein, dairy or non-dairy alternatives, and fats. While kids may not always choose to eat all the food groups available, the example is there for them to learn by watching you, and they eventually pick up on the habit.

Balanced Meals	
Instead of...	*Try...*
• A snack of crackers	• Crackers, cheese and apples
• A snack of yogurt	• Yogurt, chopped nuts, berries
• A lunch of sandwich and chips	• Sandwich with vegetables and hummus for dipping and fruit salad

In Principle 2 we touched on the importance of your family's "food culture," which certainly applies here. In her book, *Discover Mindful Eating for Kids,* Megrette Fletcher explains it this way:

This complex relationship between food, eating and nourishment becomes a 'culture'. As families grow, this culture and common food choices fades away to become a series of invisible habits. Every family and childcare center has a food culture that is unique.[17]

Consider the type of food culture you want in your home. Then ask yourself if there's a discrepancy between the food culture you desire and the one you currently have. Now is a good time to intentionally choose which foods and meal traditions you want to nourish your family.

Teaching Nutrition at Different Stages

I've listed nutrition education by age to see how it gradually builds overtime. Of course, the recommendations for the younger child can also be a good place to start for the older child. Either way, make sure you keep talk about nutrition positive so your child develops a rewarding relationship with healthy habits.

Infancy to Preschool

Use teachable moments

The food habits children are building are by far the most important education they get! Enhance these daily interactions with little tidbits of information. Your child asks for the same food they had yesterday? Let them know *we don't eat the same things every day (message: we eat a variety of food).* Your child wants to eat when he is bored? Let him know *snack time is an hour away so let's do something else (message: we don't eat when bored).*

I call this the "no with the why," explaining why you aren't doing something so they learn too.

Focus on frequency

Your child wants another treat when they already had ice cream earlier? Let her know *you already had something sweet today so let's skip it and have it another time.* This is teaching children that you have goodies less often but they are still enjoyable – and they will get them again.

Teach food before nutrition

The more kids experience and learn about food the better. Later, what they learn about nutrition will be in line with what is familiar. In my book, *What to Cook for Dinner with Kids,* I show how to give kids small cooking jobs for every meal. Be sure to take them with you to the grocery, farmer's market, and different restaurants. Always explain about the type of food present so they are always learning.

Make the taste and satisfaction connection

Show children that foods like fruits and vegetables are satisfying and tasty. Make them lots of different ways – as a side dish, roasted, salad, in smoothies, and in muffins. Don't give extra attention like saying "this is healthy because it has X." Just serve it in a tasty way like you do other foods. And don't sneak! Kids benefit from seeing what goes into the food they are eating, and when you aren't honest with them it can degrade trust.

School-Age

Help children see the connection between eating and meaningful activities

When you can, point out the connection between food and meaningful activities. Kids that play soccer will have more energy to run if they eat a balanced meal before game time (*I know you want chips, but to have energy for your game, a sandwich with some fruit is better*). If they typically have trouble focusing on homework, help them see how different foods can help their concentration (*I know you want chips but something with more food groups, including protein, will help you focus better. Why don't I use the leftover chicken from dinner last night to make you a quesadilla?*).

Try to keep this truthful without exaggerating benefits. If a child is told she will grow big and strong from eating veggies and sees she is no stronger or taller after a while, she won't believe such statements. Worse yet, she'll figure out that "these foods are so bad mommy and daddy have to lie about the benefits to get me to eat it!"

Teach more about food

As kids get older, you can build on your food teaching by explaining the different food groups and how you put together balanced meals and snacks. Slowly allow them to start making a snack or packed lunch with your guidance. This is also a good time to teach specific skills in the kitchen instead of them just helping.

Expand on their nutrition questions

Children are the most interested when they ask questions about nutrition, which inspires learning. Be sure not to blow off these questions but to take time to sit them down and explain things. Also, ask them to share what they learn at school, even if it's just a friend offering up nutrition advice. Because what they learn in the outside world may not be in line with what you want to teach them.

Teenage Years

Give them more cooking responsibility

In the later teen years, parents need to think about how children will do on their own with food. Pick a night each week when they can choose a meal and make it from start to finish, getting all the ingredients, too. This is great practice for when they are away at college or out on their own. Even if children stay at home, they should contribute by making meals.

Get specific about nutrition

Think of everything you do in regards to food and teach it to your teen. Whether it's reading labels, gathering credible nutrition information, saving recipes, or grocery shopping, be sure they are well versed on these topics before they leave home.

Developmentally Appropriate Nutrition

The goal with nutrition education is to provide *just enough* information in developmentally appropriate ways, until a child is ready to be on their own. Too much, you risk misinterpretation and eventual burnout. Too little, and you have missed opportunities to build positive connections to nutritious foods and physical activity.

Make Nutrition a Rewarding Part of Eating Summary

Every parent will have their own style when it comes to teaching nutrition and health. And no doubt every child reacts in a unique way. There are just so many people who have a negative and conflicting view of nutrition. Your goal is to make it a rewarding part of eating, one that adds to life, not takes away from it. Here are the key takeaways from Principle 4:

1) Avoid eating rules at the table, harping on which foods are healthy and unhealthy, and focusing on the negatives of eating goodies.
2) Keep nutrition positive by finding tasty ways to make nutritious items, helping kids make the connection between food and how they feel, and explaining the roles different foods have.

3) Give children hands-on experience with food such as helping in the kitchen, picking out items at the store, or making their own snack with guidance from you.

4) Be conscious about the food you expose children to on a daily basis as it makes up your family's food culture. Serve balanced meals that help increase satisfaction and nutrition variety.

5) Based on a child's age and development, educate them about nutrition whether it's explaining why you're saying no to food for a toddler, answering nutrition questions for your school-age child, or reviewing labels with a teen.

Now that we've covered the positives about nutrition, we need to focus on the pleasure of meals, because that takes everything we've talked about up to the next level.

PRINCIPLE 5

PUT PLEASURE AT THE CENTER OF YOUR TABLE

"When the joy goes out of eating, nutrition suffers."
–Ellyn Satter

Anna makes sure meals in her house get special treatment. Her family eats together at the dining room table at dinnertime. For dinner, she sets the table which includes a nice tablecloth and a candle. Her family says grace before eating and her son usually adds "Thank you God for this food." When she and her son have lunch together, she puts on some relaxing music to listen to.

While these are small things, they all work toward making eating a more enjoyable experience. Research shows eating pleasure boosts enjoyment as well as nutrition. Often, we forget in our attempts to get meals on the table and get kids fed, that the atmosphere we create around eating is important.

Pleasure is an important but overlooked part of raising a

mindful eater. Too often, food pleasure is paired with gluttony while in other countries like France "enjoy your food" is worked into dietary guidelines. When you think about it, people who abuse food don't take the time to enjoy it enough. So let's dig a bit deeper into the role pleasure at the table plays in your child's emerging relationship with food.

<u>The Food Framework – Health Before Enjoyment</u>

Gina wanted family meals to be enjoyable, but in her pursuit of getting meals on the table pleasure felt like a luxury she couldn't afford. First, was her children's behavior – they were constantly acting up so she disciplined them, sometimes ordering them to their room. Then they always seemed to take the starchy food first, wanting to skip the protein and veggies. She was constantly devising ways to get them to eat the healthy food, which was exhausting.

The truth was no one enjoyed dinnertime. Her kids were starting to associate dread with eating together as a family. They often left the table dissatisfied, even the rare times their eating performance pleased their parents. Inside Gina's children was a growing sense of guilt for wanting the wrong food, and always disappointing their parents. Eating out was everyone's refuge.

The wonderful food that Gina went to the trouble of making was going to waste but not because the kids barely ate it. It was because the whole experience was wrapped up in negativity. The kids were not exploring food or tuning into hunger and fullness, and their relationship with food was at risk. They just wanted to get their "duty" of eating over with.

The Negative Food Environment

Research suggests that the when the atmosphere around food is negative, children don't eat as well.[1] In one study, a more disapproving food environment such as hostility and inconsistent discipline was linked to more overweight and obesity than a warm and responsive family table.[2] A strong inverse relationship between eating enjoyment and picky eating has been found, meaning that the more food is enjoyed, the less picky the kids are.[3] Controlled eating atmospheres filled with pressure and restriction, researchers believe, can hinder a child's eating.

One of the factors that kills family meal joy is the constant pressure to get kids to eat a certain way. Many times, parents are reacting to a child who is more difficult to feed, whether it's pickiness or a big eater. Children experience different texture and taste worlds, which is why using force and pressure tends to make everything worse.

Most families don't realize decreased enjoyment may also result in poor digestion and absorption of nutrients. Take a study where women were given Thai food. Women who claimed the Thai meal was too spicy, thus enjoying it less, absorbed 50 percent less iron than the women who enjoyed the spicy meal. When the meal was pureed into mush to be less desirable, it decreased iron absorption by 70 percent![4] This has to do with the anticipatory part of digestion called the cephalic phase, the foreplay for eating. Digestion doesn't just occur when food hits the gastroinestinal tract, but rather it begins before the meal with anticipation of seeing food, smelling it, and developing an appetite. This prepares the body to digest food by stimulating saliva, gastric acid in the stomach, and pancreatic secretions like insulin. This "gearing up" of physiological processes intensifies the more a food is liked or wanted but that is diminished when eating it is anticipated to be a non-pleasurable experience.[5]

Food enjoyment and pleasure are important building blocks of health and nutrition. While I understand how tempting it can be to "get kids to eat," it's not worth the risk of making eating a negative experience for the child.

Desire & Habits

The concept of developing healthy habits in young children is very popular. The idea is if kids can continually participate in a positive habit when they are young, they will unconsciously do it when they get older. For certain activities like brushing teeth and making your bed, this certainly applies. But what about more complex activities? Consider a habit that was unpleasant or you were forced to do as a child. Do you partake in it now? For some, it might be going to church, eating certain foods, or visiting certain places. Odds are, if you don't desire to repeat this action as an adult, the habit became unstuck.

In his book *The Biology of Desire,* Marc Lewis, PhD, explains how it's the experiences that get repeated most often that actually change synapses in the brain to form habits. But there's a special ingredient for this to happen: *desire.* In fact, he explains that desire is evolution's agent for getting us to pursue goals repeatedly. Desire is the emotional state that propels learning.[6]

Consider what happens when healthy food is forced in the name of making it a habit. In one study of more than 100 college students, out of those who experienced forced-food consumption as a child, 72 percent said they would not now, as an adult, eat the food they were forced to eat as a child. Being made to eat resulted in feelings of conflict, with 31 percent experiencing strong conflict, 41 percent moderate conflict and 29 percent slight conflict. Forty-nine percent said they cried, 55 percent experienced nausea, and 20 percent vomited.[7] Most of the responses to the experience were negative with feelings of anger, fear, disgust, confusion, and humiliation.

So making kids eat food before they are ready can actually work to make it an anti-habit. Of course, a small percentage of these college students said being made to eat opened them up to new foods, but they were in the minority. Encouragement and food modeling have been found to be more effective than making a child eat. Remember, that once negative associations to food are planted, they can continue to grow for a lifetime. Instead, you want to plant the seeds of desire.

The Mindful Framework – Enjoyment Before Health

Once Gina switched to a Mindful Framework, she could see that the lack of enjoyment at dinner was working against her kids' eating. She also realized that she didn't grow up in a family where meals were pleasurable, so she was lacking good role models. She gave it a try by letting her children know they no longer needed to eat a certain way but she did want them to get involved with meals. She shared weekly meal plans for input and assigned small jobs for dinner. She also made sure there was something each of her kids accepted at the table, so she didn't have to worry they would go hungry. They started rituals like saying thanks for the meal and her daughter enjoyed setting the table to look nice. Once the meal was on the table, she and her husband focused on conversing and connecting with the kids, not pointing out what they were or weren't eating.

At first, Gina was disappointed in how her children ate, but she liked that the meals were actually more pleasant, so she focused on that. Over time, things began to improve and she noticed her children coming willingly to the table, often choosing to stay when they were done eating, and slowly began to explore new foods. They were more calm when eating and the process was more rewarding for everyone.

Most importantly, sharing meals as a family was becoming linked to connection, good times, and enjoyment.

Why Nutrition and Pleasure go Together

We have a narrative in society that portrays pleasure of eating as a problem. A study in the journal *Appetite* describes this as "visceral eating pleasure," something that must be controlled or suppressed even at the cost of a person's well-being. Triggers for visceral eating pleasure are typically based on environmental cues (external eating) and internal emotions (emotional eating). On the flip side is "epicurean eating pleasure," which views pleasure and eating as one in the same with moderation and well-being. This type of eating focuses on the sensory aspect of food and evaluation of food's meaning that is largely in people's control.[8]

Let's say Joyce represents visceral eating pleasure. She sees her eating pleasures as weakness – anything chocolate, salty food like chips, and most foods with sugar sends her off track. She is a restrained eater who successfully eats healthy, smallish portions most of the time, but when her favorite foods are available or she gets stressed, she breaks from her healthy routine. She is pretty good about getting back on track but the effort to control her cravings takes up a lot of mental space.

Now you have Jane, who takes great pleasure in the

experience of eating. She plans her meals and always sits down to enjoy them, often making her eating place pleasant. She enjoys the whole experience of eating from the anticipation, to the smell, to the feel of food in her mouth. She is sure to include all the foods she enjoys from chocolate to veggies. She doesn't need to eat a lot to be satisfied and feels food adds great value to her life, contributing to her happiness.

The eating experience of Jane, which exemplifies Epicurean eating pleasure, is linked not just to smaller portion size by choice, but feelings of well-being. Even though both Jane and Joyce eat similar nutritious diets, Jane is likely healthier because of her enhanced feelings of well-being and true food enjoyment. It takes a lot of energy to resist food and then feel guilty for eating it. In our food-centric environment, Epicurean eating pleasure makes more sense. You don't have to be a foodie either, you just need to embrace food in a positive way. The researchers of the *Appetite* study, sum it up this way:

This focus on the visceral aspect of eating pleasures gave rise to the belief that eating moderation must be externally imposed on our pleasure-seeking bodies through strict moral guidelines about what is "right" and "wrong" to eat... To contrast, the Epicurean perspective suggests that pleasure may in fact facilitate moderation and wellbeing. For this reason some researchers advocate a paradigm shift from "food as health" to "food as wellbeing," and call for research to give a more holistic and positive role to taking pleasure in food.

This is the type of eating pleasure we can teach our kids. Not just going on about nutrition and health, but the sensory quality of food. We can start traditions and rituals as discussed in the next section. The more pleasure children get from the eating experience, the better. Pleasure may very well be the missing component of raising a mindful eater.

Rituals & Gratitude

Harvard researchers performed four experiments to examine the effect of rituals on enjoyment of food (chocolate, lemonade, and carrots). In every experiment, rituals heightened eating enjoyment. In the first experiment, half the subjects in the chocolate experiment were asked to break the chocolate bar in half without unwrapping and then unwrap and eat half of it. After that, they could unwrap the second part and eat it. Compared to the group not asked to perform the ritual, the ritual group reported more flavor and savoring of the chocolate.[9]

Whether it's setting the table, saying grace, tossing the salad, the order in which meals are served, or anything your family regularly does with mealtime, rituals are likely to increase food's pleasure and the value of food for every family member. According to the study, rituals are beneficial in a variety of ways:

...families that consistently enact ritual behaviors have children with better self-control and academic performance than families that do not make use of rituals. This suggests that perhaps enacting rituals around food as a family would not only heighten the consumption experience but lead to more broadly positive outcomes.

Another way to increase pleasure with meals is to focus on gratitude, which has been shown to positively affect well-being.[10] In one study of 221 early adolescents, those who were asked to regularly count their blessings in class reported significantly higher satisfaction with school three weeks later.[11]

There are a variety of ways to plant the seed of gratitude when it comes to food. First, incorporate the ritual of expressing gratitude for the meal, whether it's a prayer or just giving thanks. Second, enforce a "no complaining" rule at meals, encouraging kids to focus on the positive at mealtime. And last, visiting farms, farmer's markets, or growing your own food will help children feel more connected to what they are eating.

Family Activities

There are lots of ways we can teach children to appreciate and enjoy food. Here are some specific examples that come to mind.

Tactile play

In a study out of the UK, two- to five-year-olds were engaged in tactile play with sticky foods such as mashed potatoes. The children who enjoyed this tactile play had lower rates of food neophobia (fear of new food).[12] There is a lot that can be learned by noticing and touching food to understand its unique qualities.

Start a food journey with your kids introducing food groups and helping them link each group with the five senses. Grains can be sticky (think rice), dense (breads), or crispy (crackers). Vegetables can take on all sorts of sensory qualities depending on how they are prepared. Raw veggies are crunchy but so are roasted veggies except they are soft on the inside. When you put veggies in soups or sauces, they often take the flavor of the dish, but they also add texture.

The idea is to get kids involved as much as possible with

different foods and how they feel, smell, look (color), and how that transcends to the eating experience. This gives children a wider range of experience with food beyond just taste and the sensory items they are drawn to.

Explore the five tastes

There are some tastes kids take longer to appreciate such as bitter and sour. By exploring food and different tastes, kids and adults can learn a lot.

Take the five tastes (sweet, sour, salty, bitter, and savory) and have kids place pictures of food that matches on a paper, while having a few foods available for touching and tasting. For example, show the difference between sweet fruit and a sweet drink or candy. And while sour isn't always pleasing, mixing a sour food with other ingredients can change its taste profile like adding sugar to lemon juice to make lemonade. Some vegetables may taste bitter plain but when paired with a dressing or after roasting, the taste changes.

Traditions at the table

There are all sorts of rituals that can be started at the table from saying grace to helping with the meal to sharing stories. If you want to start some new rituals ask your kids for input. Maybe you have a list of topics for dinner in a bowl and someone gets to pick one at each dinner. One may be telling your high and low point of the day or another is sharing something about yourself you don't think the family knows.

If you haven't already, be sure to add traditions around food during the holidays or special occasions. Children benefit most from rituals when they are involved in them, versus just watching others.

Family-style meals

As mentioned in Principle 2, I recommend family-style meals, placing bowls of food on the table and pass around allowing everyone to take some. Although parents are still in charge of the menu, children get some ownership and autonomy by serving themselves (instead of a pre-plated meal). It's a very peaceful and enjoyable way to share a meal as a family.

Put Pleasure at the Center of Your Table Summary

There's little doubt that enjoying meals is an integral part of raising kids with a healthy relationship to food. Why is this so hard? I think it's our cultural tendency to ensure eating is all about making the right choices. But remember, desire is what leads to the habit of making good food choices, not a sense of guilt or obligation. And focusing on pleasure also means better nutrient absorption, more care taken in planning meals, and prioritizing quality over quantity.

Here's a quick summary of how to put pleasure at the center of your table:

1) Plan and schedule family meals, asking family members for input, and make sure there's something at the table each person likes.
2) Create rituals and traditions at family meals, including special meals during holidays. Get children directly involved with these rituals.
3) Invite children to help with meal preparation and

setting the table.

4) At mealtime, focus on connection and conversation instead of what and how much children eat. Serve meals family style and allow each person to serve himself or herself.

5) Take time out from meals to explore the texture and taste of food. Educate kids about how different foods feel and taste, and about the art of putting a balanced meal together.

With some effort, meal enjoyment can improve greatly, and so will the health and well-being of every family member. Next, zeroing in on how children feel about their bodies, a vitally important aspect of raising a mindful eater.

PRINCIPLE 6

TEACH BODY APPRECIATION

"Take care of your body as if you were going to live forever; and take care of your soul as if you were going to die tomorrow." –St. Augustine

Angela grew up thinking that constant vigilance around eating was normal. After all, her mom was always dieting and she joined her at age twelve. After getting married, Angela had so little body fat she stopped getting her periods and couldn't get pregnant. She was told she needed to gain weight and began to struggle with binge-eating. After gaining 40 pounds and stopping exercise, she was finally able to become pregnant. But this left her with a body that felt unrecognizable.

During her pregnancy, Angela stumbled upon *Intuitive Eating* and slowly began the process of listening to and appreciating her body. Once she felt comfortable on her new path, she saw nothing positive about her previous way of relating to food, "Diets haven't done anything good for me," she pointed out.

She is committed to passing down a healthy relationship with food and body image to her two-year-old daughter. That being said, her daughter is 98 percentile for weight and is already getting comments from other people about being chubby. She feels there is so much misinformation out there about weight. Don't raise a child to be overweight, but don't restrict them or mention weight. What's a parent to do?

Angela's right, there's not enough clear advice on the tough topic of size, weight, and body shape for families. There are so many harmful messages our kids receive – and potential teasing – that we need to help prepare them. Because how your child comes to view his or her body, and the bodies of those around them, is a vital piece of the puzzle. Let's start by examining how seeing weight through Food Framework leaves us with more questions than answers.

The Food Framework – Fix Your Body with Food

Tina had two kids, a daughter and a son. She worried most about her nine-year-old daughter, Hayley, because she had always been larger than average. In fourth grade, Hayley started to compare her body to her peers and asked her mom about it. Tina always responded with "you're fine," knowing that talking about weight wasn't a good thing.

While they were at the park, a young boy called Hayley "fat girl," and that was the breaking point. When they got home, Tina couldn't hold back anymore, as she felt her daughter's self-esteem was on the line. She told her daughter they needed to do something about her weight or else this would keep happening, and her health was at risk.

In the emotional turmoil, Hayley agreed, never wanting to feel this kind of shame again.

Once her mom acknowledged her weight as a problem, it confirmed what Hayley had been considering recently: her body was all wrong. They sought help and started eating healthier. Tina noticed her daughter slimming down but then there were parties and sleepovers where she would sneak food. Hayley always felt guilty and never told her mom. These feelings of shame and guilt around food – and reminders of the fight with her body – drove her to emotional eating. She engaged in a disordered eating cycle that would stick for years to come: eat healthy/small portions, slim down, and then eventually binge and gain weight again.

Dissatisfied Bodies: Dieting & Disordered Eating

According to a 2016 report from the American Academy of Pediatrics, half of teenage girls and one quarter of boys are dissatisfied with their bodies. Body dissatisfaction has adverse effects as stated in the report:

Body dissatisfaction is a known risk factor for both eating disorders and disordered eating: higher scores of body dissatisfaction are associated with more dieting and unhealthy weight-control behaviors in both boys and girls, reduced physical activity in girls, and more binge eating in boys.[1]

The Food Framework goes something like this: if you don't like the way your body looks, you can change it with limiting food. This is why body dissatisfaction in both children and adults leads to unhealthy weight control practices.[2,3] This, researchers believe, predispose people to a greater risk of weight gain. It's not just heavier kids at risk. Something called "body weight misperception" – seeing yourself as overweight even when you're not – is common in adolescence. In one study, adolescent girls of normal weight who perceived themselves as overweight were 30 percent more likely to become obese twelve years later.[4] The boys were 89 percent more likely to become obese in adulthood. It's not just children who worry about their weight but parents, too. When parents perceive their children as overweight, their children are more likely to gain weight over time.[5]

There's an important difference between normal eating, disordered eating, and eating disorders. According to Eating Disorders Victoria, normal eating varies from person to person but ultimately comes down to a positive relationship with food.[6] Some days normal eaters may eat less and other days more, for instance, but they don't get caught up labeling foods as good or bad, obsessing over sweets, and they treat food as just one component of a healthy life. This is different from disordered eating, which interferes with all aspects of well-being and may include dieting, binge-eating, skipping meals, obtaining self-worth from body shape, and chronic restricting. People are at risk for disordered eating when they become dissatisfied with their body or want to lose weight. Disordered eating increases the risk of developing an eating disorder. In fact, one study showed that kids with the most restrictive diets were eighteen times more likely to develop an eating disorder.[7] Eating disorders, such as anorexia, bulimia, and binge-eating disorder, are extreme eating behaviors as defined in Table P6.1. If you suspect an eating disorder, don't delay getting your child help as early treatment improves outcomes.

Table P6.1 The Eating Spectrum

Eating Type	What is it?	What parents can do
Normal	Positive relationship with food; eats balanced meals without feeling guilty or obsessing about always eating healthy	Watch for signs of body dissatisfaction that can turn a normal eater into a disordered eater
Disordered Eating	Decreased quality of life due to one or more of the following: dieting, binge-eating, mindlessly eating, skipping meals, seeking happiness from body shape and restricting food	Work to get a child back to normal eating either through changes to feeding, discussions, modeling, or professional help
Eating Disorders	*Anorexia:* restricts food despite low weight; intense fear of gaining weight; distorted body image *Bulimia:* Eats large amounts of food followed by vomiting or other medications; self-worth tied to body shape *Binge-Eating:* Episodes of eating large quantities of food and feeling badly afterwards	Get professional help ASAP if you see any of the warning signs: • eats very little food • skips meals • compulsive exercise • unexplained weight loss • use of diet pills or laxatives • self-induced vomiting • social isolation • fear of gaining weight

Stigma & Shame

Body dissatisfaction doesn't come out of nowhere, it comes from our anti-fat culture. This biased news and entertainment propaganda comes to us at lightning speed, and although the news media base their reports on scientific studies, they often dramatize it with words like "war" and "epidemic." The news media is also more likely than science to blame individuals for their weight.[8] The entertainment media is no better. In a review of primetime shows, it was common for overweight women to be teased by men, followed by audience laughter. Obese individuals are often shown overeating junk food, living unhappy lives, and are seen as being uninvolved with life. Children's shows often portray big kids as disliked and of poor character like Harry Potter's greedy and mean cousin Dudley.[9]

The saddest part is kids have picked up on the anti-fat culture. The most common reason for bullying in schools isn't race, religion, or sexual orientation, it's body weight.[10] According to one study, more than 90 percent of adolescents have witnessed their peers being bullied due to excess weight. And of those overweight youth seeking treatment, 70 percent said their friends and peers have teased them as well as a significant number of adults – PE teachers/coaches (42 percent), parents (37 percent) and teachers (27 percent).[11]

A 2012 report, "Weight Bias: A Social Justice Issue" from the Rudd Center for Food Policy and Obesity at Yale University, details how weight stigma decreases academic performance and increases risk of depression, poor body image, suicidal thoughts, and unhealthy habits such as dieting and decreased physical activity.[10] Not only that, people who experience weight stigma are also more likely to gain weight – or stay obese – over time.[12]

"There is a misconception that individuals can be shamed into losing weight (our culture does it constantly, think of the Biggest Loser)," said Tracy Tylka, introduced earlier in the book. "Individuals who experience weight stigma internalize this stigma and think badly of themselves, which then lowers their tendency to appreciate their bodies, increases their eating in the absence of hunger, which then lowers physical and psychological health."

Stigma and shame around body shape and size simply doesn't work. But luckily there is another way, and it starts with teaching all kids to appreciate their bodies.

The Mindful Framework – Body Appreciation

Let's see what happens when Tina switches to a Mindful Framework. After the boy at the park teased her daughter about her weight, she comforted Hayley and didn't say much at all. Instead, she got some help to decide once and for all if her child's weight was a problem. First, she examined her daughter's growth chart and could see that she stayed at about the same curve her whole life. This, she was told, signals her body's genetic blueprint and not problematic accelerated growth. She also looked at what and how she was feeding her daughter. Hayley ate balanced meals at regular times, didn't graze in between meals, and she had sweets a few times a week. Although she had a hearty appetite, Hayley seemed to have a healthy relationship with food in that she didn't fixate on sweets or ask for food much between meals.

The most pressing issue was her daughter's social comparisons. She had started noticing her body looked different than her friends and had already reached out to her mom for reassurance. Tina got a plan on how she could talk to her daughter about her body. But first, Tina had to confront her own issues. The truth was she was frightened to raise a child that didn't fit the healthy norm as she was naturally small-framed while her husband was bigger like her daughter. Just acknowledging this bias helped, and Tina was able to let go of this dreamed-up idea she had of what growing up healthy meant.

Tina started with the boy at the park and what he said, asking Hayley to share what she was feeling. They talked about how people tend to make fun of the things they don't understand, and what she can do if that happens again. She explained how society is not always accepting of different body sizes, and that's wrong. Through frequent conversations like this they talked about accepting the body you are born with, understanding that looks are only one small part of who you are, and that healthy habits keep your body strong and healthy. Tina also educated her daughter and son about attitudes that make people feel bad about their bodies. She pointed out unrealistic media images, unproductive messages about food, and together they resisted unhealthy norms about weight.

Body Appreciation = Self-care

Unlike body dissatisfaction, children who feel good about their bodies are more likely to maintain healthy, sustainable habits.[1] Research also suggests that *perceived body acceptance* by others is important in how children come to view their bodies. So the family culture around weight and whether a child feels accepted is a key part of the puzzle.[13] "This is what we do know is helpful: everyone, regardless of their size, can benefit from taking good care of their body and learning to look at it with love and appreciation," said Linda Bacon PhD, introduced earlier in the book. "Start there. You'll feel better about yourself, which is really what kids are really looking for when they want to lose weight."

The definition of body appreciation, according to Tracy Tylka is "holding favorable opinions toward the body regardless of its appearance, accepting the body along with its deviations from societal beauty ideals, respecting the body by attending to its needs and engaging in healthy behaviors, and protecting the body by rejecting unrealistic media appearance ideals." Body appreciation is about having a deep and respectful relationship with your body. Although society encourages an aesthetic view, parents can help kids view their bodies more holistically.

A positive body image helps kids in a variety of ways. First, it helps protect children from the constant negative media exposure they get.[14] Second, a positive body image has been linked to better self-esteem and well-being.[15] Third, children are more likely to be intuitive eaters. "Based on a study in *Developmental Psychology*, we do know that initial levels of body appreciation predict future levels of intuitive eating one year later," said Tylka. "Appreciating the body helps individuals stay in tune with the body's needs and respect the body, which facilitates their attention to their hunger and satiety cues (intuitive eating) and following these cues to respect their bodies."[16]

Kathy Kater, psychotherapist and author of *Healthy Bodies: Teaching Kids What They Need to Know*, created The Healthy Body Image Curriculum to help young children (fourth through sixth grade) view their bodies in a positive light and decrease their risk of eating disorders.[17] The curriculum focuses on everything from the biology of size and shape to decoding media images. Kater's research shows that educating children in this way is beneficial, especially before the middle-school years, a time when body dissatisfaction and dieting can take root. This curriculum is based on three important components: understanding what you cannot change; taking control of what you can; and learning to critically think about size issues. Let's take a look.

Understanding What You Cannot Change

The first component of the Healthy Body Image Curriculum is aimed at helping children understand what is happening to their body during growth and development. First are the normal changes that occur during puberty that often result in "temporary out-of-proportion growth." This means that (girls in particular) often gain extra fat before they grow in height. Next is genetics that determine someone's frame and limits the ability to alter their shape through dietary means. In fact, restriction or ignoring hunger works against the body growing and developing the way nature intended. Trying to change basic biology – size, shape, weight, and hunger – is an uphill battle.

If you, like Tina, are concerned about your child's weight, you can check your child's weight trajectory to see if their growth is problematic. This can be done by getting copies of your child's growth chart and looking for trends. Pediatric dietitian Katie Mulligan explains it this way:

Whether children fall at the 50th, or 95th percentile isn't necessarily a concern of mine, if that's where they've always trended. Childhood overweight and obesity become a problem when children grow "off their curve." This is when kids follow a nice line on their growth chart for a few years, but then begin to trail upwards into the area of the growth chart where there aren't any lines to follow. They may also be jumping percentile lines, which means they go from the 75th percentile to the 90th to the 110th and so on. The concern comes when they "jump percentiles" several years in a row; not for just one year and then settle back into their curve.

In Principle 3, we mention Dara-Lynn Weiss's book *The Heavy,* which chronicles how she put her seven-year-old daughter on a weight-loss diet. While reading the story of her child (Bea), it was apparent that Bea's growth had skyrocketed up from her typical growth pattern which is indeed a red flag. But instead of using a Mindful Framework to consider root causes, Weiss focused on food and restriction. Worse yet, you could see how keeping her child on a diet put a strain on the mother-daughter relationship (see Principle 8 for why this is important).

Is weight loss always bad? Not necessarily. When changes are made that get to the root cause of unnecessary weight gain, a child may lose some weight or stay the same as he grows. This is different from dieting which includes restricting and ignoring hunger and satiety for the goal of losing weight (for example, the child eats a small portion at dinner and doesn't eat more even when hungry). If your child has been growing fast, I recommend seeking professional help. Families in these cases need all the help and support they can get. See the resource section at the end of the book.

Although you can't control the weight and shape of your child's body, you can do your part in making the home environment conducive to healthy and balanced habits that can last a lifetime.

Understanding What You Can Change

The second part of The Healthy Body Image Curriculum teaches children to focus on what is in their control. First is how children view themselves. Children learn that looks are only one aspect of who they are, and it pays to invest in other areas for a rich and rewarding life. These are qualities like being kind, developing talents, and being a good friend to others. The key is to encourage kids to share their true self with the world and not spend their energy trying to live up to some unrealistic ideal.

Next are the healthy habits that further enrich a rewarding life, discussed throughout this book. Eating balanced meals and satisfying hunger, for example, provides lasting energy and helps kids stay focused during the day. Being physically active also promotes energy and keeps children feeling good and sleeping well. Much of these self-care habits are stressed in Principle 7, but the key is to focus on what a child can control (healthy habits) versus what they can't (the body they were born with).

Even when well-intentioned "weight talk" in families such as comments about a child's, parent's or anyone else's weight, can be counterproductive. One example might be putting down your own body or commenting how someone else has gained or lost weight. A 2016 report from the Academy of Pediatrics summarizes the research:

Several studies have found that parental weight talk, whether it involves encouraging their children to diet or talking about their own dieting, is linked to overweight...However, if the focus of the conversation was only on healthful eating behaviors, overweight adolescents were less likely to diet and use unhealthy weight control practices.[1]

Experts across the board agree that weight should be de-emphasized in favor of healthy behaviors. This is true for kids of all shapes and sizes.

Teach Critical Thinking

One of the biggest myths is that parents should never talk about weight with their child. I'm not referring to the weight talk just mentioned but having meaningful and ongoing conversations about size diversity. The goal is to teach kids how to critically think about the complex food and weight culture in which we live. This is the third – and very important – component of the Healthy Body Image Curriculum.

Take the results of an internet survey with bullied teens at the Youth Voice Project. The most helpful coping mechanism adolescents used to deal with bullying was to think differently about what happened. It was the teens who understood they were not to blame for what happened and that it showed more about the person doing the bullying. According to the site, "Many students in our survey said they realized that the people who were doing mean things to them were acting immature."[18] This is very different from a young person internalizing bullying by believing something is wrong with them.

Linda Bacon provides insight on how to broach this subject with kids: "It makes sense that kids would be concerned about being fat in this anti-fat culture, and I think it's important to honor these fears. Telling them what we know to be true – that weight stigma is wrong and kids can be beautiful and healthy at every size – isn't enough to help them change their attitude and behavior, when they can see the real rewards people get for being thinner in this culture. It's important to be real with them, and acknowledge that."

As Bacon suggests, having honest discussions with your child about society's distorted view of size will help them to start to question it. Many people don't understand that people come in all shapes and sizes and that size doesn't tell you anything about what or even how much a person eats, and it reveals absolutely nothing about character.

"I like to use the analogy of skin color. Sure, we know that white people often get treated better because of their lighter skin, but we don't suggest that black people bleach their skin as a solution," said Bacon. "We recognize that bleaching may be harmful, may not work, and doesn't get at the real problem: racism. Nor will trying to lose weight. Dieting isn't effective and it just makes people feel bad about their eating."

In addition to teaching kids about weight diversity is teaching them about the media's portrayal of the Thin Ideal. "Research with kids as young as three-to-five years of age reveals that they show signs of adopting the belief that goodness in females was related to thinness," said Jennifer Shewmaker, PhD, author of *Sexualized Media Messages and Our Children: Teaching Kids to Be Smart Critics and Consumers*. "But it's important to remember that there are variables in their personal life, such as family and community, that can help them process media messages and choose a healthy response." Shewmaker provides the following tips to parents:

Talk with your child

When you see examples of females being presented as valuable primarily for their appearance or of goodness equated with thinness or muscularity for boys, point it out and open the door for ongoing conversation. Address "fear of fat" directly when it comes up.

Monitor your child's media and product use

Is your child receiving a lot of messages about the importance of how they look? You may choose to restrict their exposure to certain shows or products, or you may choose to allow it, but only with your active participation. You can guide your children in developing the ability to critique media messages by doing so yourself. Then prompt them to do so as well.

Build community

To challenge the idea that how a person looks is the most important thing about her, it is very important to have a community of support that also promotes other characteristics as valuable. Find other parents, families, and groups that will support your child as they reject and challenge unhealthy ideas.

Just think, the more families discuss these hard issues, the healthier and happier kids will be. They will no longer be victims of a society that promotes unhealthy norms about weight, because they will have learned the skills for rejecting it and being comfortable in their own bodies.

Is the Answer to Shame Self-Esteem or Self-Compassion?

In a study published in *PLoS ONE*, 25 parents and grandparents revealed their experience with body image growing up. There were a variety of experiences like one participant still living with the painful comments about her weight by her parents, "I carry that with me today. I still think of that...That's why it's so important to me not to make an issue out of weight, because those comments last forever and ever." Another participant said, "I don't think I've ever liked my body weight, even though I was only a size five up until I was eighteen, and that's fairly small, but I never liked myself." No matter what was said, none of the participants – regardless of size – described their emerging childhood body image in positive terms. The central theme was a universal feeling of shame for falling short of society's ideals. And even more sadly, many of the adults in the study reported that those early experiences carried over to adulthood.[19]

Brené Brown, shame researcher and best-selling author of several books including *Daring Greatly*, deftly explains the difference between shame and guilt. Guilt is how you feel when you did something you shouldn't have, separating the behavior from your value. But shame is the painful feeling that you are flawed because of who you are.

We know feeling bad about our body can instantly bring up feelings of shame. Society's attempt to fix this has been to pump people up with self-esteem. Isn't that what the before and after pictures of commercial weight-loss programs are trying to achieve? This "self-esteem culture" has some major shortcomings as pointed out by Kristin Neff PhD, author of *Self-Compassion: The Proven Power of Being Kind to Yourself*:

The main problem is that having high self-esteem requires feeling special and above average. To be called average is considered an insult in our culture. ("How did you like my performance last night?" "It was average." Ouch!) Of course, it's logically impossible for every human being on the planet to be above average at the same time. So we develop what's known as a "self-enhancement bias," which refers to the tendency to think of ourselves as superior to others on a variety of dimensions. Studies have shown that most people feel they're friendlier, more popular, funnier, nicer, more trustworthy, wiser and more intelligent than others. Ironically, most people also think they're above average in the ability to view themselves objectively! The result of wearing these rose-colored glasses isn't so pretty.[20]

Neff further explains how the self-esteem culture feeds the need to feel superior to others, which can increase social comparisons, bullying, narcissism, and being self-critical when making mistakes or not feeling like you measure up. Consider the difference between how Hayley feels when she tries to feel better about herself by slimming down versus accepting her body even when she knows it doesn't fit the ideal. In fact, social comparison is the key way that young people learn to feel badly about their bodies. Instead of trying to make a child feel good about their body by slimming down, it pays to help them develop self-compassion instead.

"Self-compassion involves being kind to ourselves when life goes awry or we notice something about ourselves we don't like, rather than being cold or harshly self-critical," Neff said on her website. "It recognizes that the human condition is imperfect, so that we feel connected to others when we fail or suffer rather than feeling separate or isolated."

Research shows that self-compassion is linked to decreased psychological distress (anxiety, depression, etc.), increased social connectedness, increased life satisfaction, and body appreciation.[21,22] One study found that self-compassion protects against what researchers call "body-related threats" such as body comparisons and getting self-esteem from appearance. In other words, the higher young women scored on self-compassion, the less likely they experienced negative effects from environmental triggers of body dissatisfaction.[23]

Self-Esteem is Not All Bad

In her book, Neff explains that there are benefits to self-esteem but the downside is that kids feel bad (or get defensive) the times they fail or fall short. This is where self-compassion comes in. It has the upside of self-esteem (feeling good about yourself), but it also helps children realize the natural dips and disappointments in life that everyone experiences.

What a relief for young people to realize they don't have to be better than others or perfect to be valued, they just need to be themselves. We all fail, make mistakes, and feel like we don't measure up at times — it's part of the human experience.

Let's Start a Revolution

In this day and age, people are hyperaware of stigmas due to race, gender, and sexual orientation. Those issues aren't behind us but they get lots of air time. Yet weight stigma does not have this type of awareness. Much of it has to do with the misconceived idea that weight is largely in someone's control, unlike other aspects like skin color, that are not.

As you and your child go into the world with this new information you will notice things you know are not good for kids. Maybe it's weighing children at school, nutrition education that demonizes food or the body, bullying from children and adults, or a pediatrician who embarrasses a child about her weight at a doctor's appointment. We know all of these things only increase weight stigma and harm the health of children, often causing scars that last a lifetime.

Be sure to ask your child to tell you what they experience in school and the outside environment. Do they notice any kids being made fun of? What's being taught in health class? An honest and open dialogue with your child will keep you abreast of what's going on, so you can speak up when appropriate. The key is to talk to others with the intent of educating them that these practices – while done with good intentions – are not good for the health and well-being of youth.

If we get enough parents and kids fighting the good fight, real change can happen, one step at a time.

Teach Body Appreciation Summary

Teaching children how to appreciate and take care of their body – no matter its size – can be a tall order. It takes dedication and a leap of faith. But the payoff – a confident and healthy child who accepts himself for who he is – is definitely worth it. This principle is not just for kids that are big, as we know this problem of body dissatisfaction occurs at all weights and sizes. And for the problem to get better, change needs to occur in everybody. Here are the main takeaways from Principle 6:

1) Understand how the Food Framework – fixing the body with food – doesn't get to root causes of eating or unnecessary weight gain and increases the risk of stigma, body dissatisfaction, eating in the absence of hunger, and dieting.
2) The first step of the Mindful Framework is to understand your child's growth trajectory by checking their growth chart. If they are indeed growing off their curve, read through all the 8 Principles to pinpoint

potential causes for the growth acceleration or get professional help.

3) Help children understand what is beyond their control, such as genetically-determined weight, shape, and appetite. Help them understand their unique growth and development and its biological and genetic roots.

4) Explain and establish the things kids can control like healthy habits that help their bodies feel good and thrive – sleep, quality food, and being active. This also includes how they view themselves and the importance of not making looks the sole purpose of their identity.

5) Teach critical thinking by explaining about weight stigma and why it's harmful. Increase awareness of anti-fat attitudes and teach media literacy.

6) Instill self-compassion in children instead of feeling like they need to always feel good about themselves. For example, being kind to yourself and others as we all face challenges and make mistakes.

Teaching body appreciation is no easy task, but it's worth every bit of effort. Next, we get into the importance of managing stress, a major barrier to raising a mindful eater.

PRINCIPLE 7

DEAL WITH STRESS EFFECTIVELY

"It's not the load that breaks you down, it's the way you carry it."–Lou Holtz

Allison was raised in a home where conflict didn't happen, or at least she didn't see it happen. As an adult, emotional upheaval was not her comfort zone. The hard part came when she had kids of her own (six, four, and two) who wear their feelings on their sleeve. She was not used to all that feeling and expressing. In fact, it was hard enough just learning how to express her feelings to her husband.

"Now as an adult, I'm learning how to do it differently with my children," she said. "The hard feelings are okay and I'm helping to create that kind of dynamic for my kids and model it for myself." Allison also started prioritizing her own sleep, rest, and diet. When she's eating well and running a few nights a week, she feels much better. She realized that what she brings into her interactions with her children influences her effectiveness as a parent.

Stress is a major player in today's families. In 2009, Dr. Robert Epstein compiled ten research-based parenting practices that produce optimal outcomes for raising children. While it was no surprise that showing love and affection topped the list, the second most important parenting practice, stress management, was a surprise. What is even more surprising is that taking steps to reduce stress was important not just for children but for adults, too. In fact, the report concluded that, *"Parents' ability to manage stress was a good predictor of the quality of their relationship with their children."[1]*

Research reveals simple ways kids and parents can learn to deal with stress more effectively. And it starts with learning some key skills. First, like we always do, let's look at what happens when we approach this challenge using the Food Framework.

The Food Framework – Manipulate Food to Improve Behavior

Joy had trouble managing her son Sam's behavior. He had difficulty sitting still and sometimes got in trouble in school for it. Sam did well academically but would always fall apart when he got home from school and wanted sweets and snack foods. In order to help him, Joy cut simple carbs from his diet, including sugar, and was sometimes successful at keeping him off gluten. Her goal was to keep Sam on a whole, no-processed-food diet to improve his behavior. When she first made the switch she saw a noticeable difference in his behavior. But over time this has lessened and she thought it had to do with his sneaking food at school and eating at his friend's house.

Joy used a reward and punishment system to motivate her son. She'd take the iPad away if he acted inappropriately, for example, or gave him extra time on the iPad if he did a chore or had a good day. Monitoring his behavior and doling out rewards and punishments took a lot of her energy but what else was she to do?

Although her son had good and bad days, the real problem left festering underneath it all: stress overload. And worst of all, her son started feeling like he could never get things right, so why even try?

Stress Before Food

Changing the quality of a child's diet can help improve behavior, but alone it's not enough to deal with the stress overload that is often lurking. "There's quite a bit of data that we have the highest stressed generation than we have ever seen," said Dr. Stuart Shanker, self-regulation expert, CEO of the MEHRIT Centre and author of *Self Reg: How to Help Your Child (and You) Break the Stress Cycle and Successfully Engage with Life.* "Many of the stressors are hidden so parents miss them."

People tend to think of stress as major events that cause hardship, instead of daily occurrences. Looking at stress as "out-of-the-norm" events means parents miss it not only in their children but in their own lives. Dr. Shanker defines stress as anything that triggers a response in the brain that requires energy. In other words, every stressor a child is faced with takes up a certain amount of energy. Potential stressors might be physiological, emotional, cognitive, social, or prosocial, according to Dr. Shanker. But all children react differently to life events. What causes stress in one child may not in another.

Let's take a child who has attention issues in school like Sam. It can take a tremendous amount of energy for these kids to sit and focus all day while other kids require much less energy to do this same task. Because much of Sam's energy is going towards sitting still and being quiet, he runs out of energy to control his impulses and gets in trouble, which only adds to his stress.

We tend to look at self-control as a strength or weakness. When it's a perceived weakness in children, parents and teachers try to drive it into kids using rewards and punishments, which Dr. Shanker says doesn't work. He explains why showcasing the classic Stanford "Marshmallow Test." In this study, researchers tell a group of four-year-olds they can have one marshmallow now or two later if they wait fifteen minutes. The kids who waited, showing more self-control, ended up being more successful later in life.[2] Dr. Shanker argues that kids who have trouble with self-control aren't weaker at all; they simply are using up too much of their energy dealing with stressors. If these kids can become self-regulated, they would exhibit self-control like their less-stressed peers. Dr. Shanker defines self-regulation as "how effectively we deal with stress and recover from it." How well we recover from different situations is the key.

Is it Food or Poor Self-regulation?

When kids experience too much stress or can't manage the stress coming their way, it negatively affects their health. Stress overload has been linked to excess weight and poor eating habits. This is because the body reacts to excess stress with hormonal, metabolic, and neural changes that can drive food intake.[3] In one study, children found to have poor self-regulation at ages three to five, had the highest BMI scores and the most rapid weight gain over nine years.[4] Another aspect of self-regulation, regulating emotions, has been linked to rapid weight gain and excess weight in middle childhood. Children who experience trouble regulating their emotions are also more likely to act out and have trouble delaying gratification.[5]

According to Dr. Shanker, signs of poor self-regulation include trouble paying attention, difficulty doing simple tasks, acting crabby in the morning, feeling unhappy during the day, being argumentative, getting angry often (this can turn violent in some children), acting highly impulsive, becoming easily distracted, having difficulty tolerating frustration, and experiencing difficulty going to bed or turning off the television/video game.

Food alone isn't going to solve this one because it's the inability to self-regulate – recover from stress – that contributes to eating habits. For instance, you can try to get a child who stays up late to eat better, but it's the lack of sleep that's fueling the food choices. Rushing to punishment makes behavior worse because it adds stress, while leaving the original stressor unaddressed. So cutting out sugar and poor eating, without dealing with underlying stress, may mean kids sneak or fight the food rules even more.

But there is another way that gets to the source, and helps kids become master self-regulators.

The Mindful Framework – Lowering and Managing Stress

When Joy applied the Mindful Framework, she stepped back to look at what was going on with Sam from a self-regulation standpoint. First, she talked to his teacher who said he does well for weeks at a time and then will have one terrible day. She had an open and honest talk with Sam, and he admitted that sitting all day is tough, as he at times wants to get up and move around, especially before taking tests. The teacher agreed to allow him to get up and move around before tests or when he's feeling agitated. Joy started taking him to the playground or letting him play outside after school before doing homework.

Next she looked at sleep, which plays a big role in self-regulation. Her son tended to go to bed too late and get up early. Together they decided on an early bedtime on school nights and Friday he could stay up an hour later. She talked to him about food and he suggested having sweets sometimes so they decided on Wednesday snack and Friday dessert. She also told him he can eat what he wants at friends' houses so there was no need to sneak. She kept nutritious food a priority – which is important for self-regulation – but was okay with providing some wiggle room.

Last was his emotions. Joy sensed he was worried a lot and decided to drop the rewards and punishments and set aside ten minutes every day for "worry time," where he could vent about what's bothering him. She couldn't believe what she was finding out! The tests at school, which picked up this year, really stressed him out. He felt he needed to always get an A to make her and his dad happy. This allowed Joy the opportunity to help him work through his anxiety and let him know that she and her husband just wanted him to learn in school, grades were not the most important thing. He also shared problems with friends and for the first time was able to release his feelings instead of keeping them pent up.

There were tremendous changes in Sam's behavior, and their relationship. This inspired Joy to work on her own ability to self-regulate, so she was making exercise and sleep a priority, saying no when she felt overwhelmed, and sharing her feelings with her husband. The whole family was self-regulating better and were happier and healthier because of it.

The Best Place to Start

Since 2007, the American Psychological Association's Stress in America Survey gauges Americans' stress levels and how it effects health and well-being. In 2014, they found that while stress levels had gone down somewhat, this didn't happen for certain populations, like parents. Parents rated stress to be an almost six out of ten, and cite money as their biggest worry. Those with the highest levels of stress were more likely to use unhealthy habits to deal with stress such as watching TV, engaging in sedentary behaviors, eating poorly, skipping meals, surfing the internet, and drinking.[6] Of course, these habits worsen stress because they further deplete resources instead of filling them back up.

Dr. Shanker encourages parents to go through the self-regulation process right along with their kids. "Parents don't self-regulate either," he said. "In fact, we are a dysregulated society!" Ultimately, he explained, children pick up on their parents' body language and self-regulation habits.

Allison, introduced in the beginning of the chapter, started going for runs after her kids went to sleep and got more shut-eye herself. She felt it helped her feel calm enough to tolerate her kids' emotions and not react to them. This is the best place to start – sleep, physical activity, and regular balanced meals – what I call the trifecta of self-care. Families that work hard to keep these three lifestyle factors in line have a head start in managing stress. When everyone is getting enough sleep and exercise, they have more energy and focus during the day. Physical activity also improves sleep quality. Regular balanced and nutritious meals fuel us throughout the day and is vital for lasting energy, improved mood, and better behavior.

A 2010 study in *Pediatrics* looked at routines and

obesity risk in 8,550 preschoolers. Researchers examined three routines: eating family meal at least five times per week, getting at least 10.5 hour of sleep a night, and getting less than two hours of daily screen time. The children who lived in homes with all three of the routines had approximately 40 percent lower risk of becoming obese compared to the children who had none of these routines. In fact, each routine by itself was associated with lower risk of obesity with all three together being the most powerful.[7] When researchers intervened and had children implement healthy routines such as sleep and watching less TV on weekdays, it led to decreased BMI.[8]

Table P7.1: Healthy Routines

Instead of...	Try..	Ask yourself...
Random use of technology	Structuring the use of screens less than two hours a day at certain times (even less on school days). Try family digital-free time after dinner.	• How do I feel when I exercise, sleep, and eat well versus when I don't? • What activities fill my energy cup during the day, and which ones take from it?
Sitting while kids play	Walking around the park or playing with children.	
Hanging around the house	Going for hikes or walks together as a family. Try after dinner in the summer and weekend mornings.	• When I'm feeling irritable, which one of these lifestyle factors is off?

| Staying up late to get things done/relax | Going to bed early and getting up to do work when you feel fresh. You can relax in the morning, too. |
| Eating at random times | Scheduling regular meals as mentioned in Principle 1. Create rituals around food (see Principle 4). |

Create family routines that help everyone benefit from the trifecta of self-care. This can go a long way to reducing or even removing stressors touched on in the next section. In addition to trying things out, ask yourself how they make you and your kids feel. Then, help kids see the connection between these habits and physical feelings. Some ideas for healthy routines are mentioned in Table P7.1.

Let's face it, taking care of ourselves with food, sleep, and activity is a smart thing to do. Of course, it can't be done every single day – and in every situation – but making self-care a priority is more than half the battle.

Identify Hidden Stressors

Helping children self-regulate begins with reframing their behavior from "this is bad, I need to punish" to understanding *why* they are acting out. Dr. Shanker points out that there's a big difference between a stress behavior and a misbehavior. So if a child is having trouble paying attention, ignoring distracters, inhibiting impulses, controlling emotions, and just not being able to stay in a calm and alert state, the potential stressors need to be examined.

Common stressors include the trifecta of self-care (too little exercise, poor sleep, and diet), family life disturbances, lack of communities, loss of parent and child connection, overexposure to screens, clutter, over-stimulation at school, and highly structured days without enough free play.

When you identify a stressor, you can work to decrease it or help the child manage it better. I know my son has trouble with noise, so we keep a quiet house, especially during homework. And too many structured activities, in addition to school, stress out my daughter, so I make an effort to ensure she gets free play time. And to be honest, sometimes I sense my kids need more one-on-one time with me or their dad when they seem to be off.

Allison found that rushing from one activity to another stressed everybody out. She'd immediately get resistance and heard, "I don't want to get my coat on," which was a trigger for her reacting. She has lessened the family schedule and now works on ways to bring her children back to calm. Take time to consider your individual stressors, as well. I have always relied heavily on the trifecta of self-care, but I realized other hidden stressors, such as clutter, screen time (especially at night), too much sitting on workdays, over committing, and not sharing my worries with others. So now I make managing these hidden stressors a priority, and when I'm feeling out of sorts, I can usually find the cause.

Another component of self-regulation, Dr. Shanker explains, is teaching kids what calm and alert feels like. This can be challenging as some children have become used to having their engine running very fast. When your child starts moving away from calm and alert, like feeling agitated, you can help her develop strategies for getting back to this state. It might be coloring, jumping on a trampoline, playing sports, free play, listening to music, or reading. It will be different for each child.

When children are calmly focused and alert, they are better able to manage their emotions, pay attention, ignore distractions, inhibit their impulses, and understand what others are thinking and feeling. They may even make better food choices. In one of Dr. Shanker's studies, once children learned to self-regulate, they began choosing fruit over sugary snacks. "Not from us telling them, the brain naturally wants quality food when it's not stressed," he said.

Emotion Coaching

Early in his career, Dr. John Gottman from the University of Illinois studied families with three-year-old children until they were fifteen. He came up with the term "meta-emotion," which is how people feel about emotion — especially difficult ones like anger. Throughout the study and observation, he made key discoveries about the impact emotional processes have on children and parents.[9]

"Much of today's popular advice to parents ignores emotion," Gottman wrote on his website. "Instead it relies on child-rearing theories that address children's misbehavior, but disregards the feelings that underlie that misbehavior. The ultimate goal of raising children should not be simply to have an obedient and compliant child. Most parents hope for much more for their children."

He found that even very loving and warm parents had trouble dealing with their child's negative emotions and the most successful parents took part in a process he calls "emotion coaching." He wrote that, "The secret to being an emotionally intelligent parent lay in how parents interacted with their children when emotions ran hot."

Children who received emotion coaching were more successful, confident, and happy than children who didn't. In fact, Gottman's research shows that children who have parents who use these techniques are better able to regulate their emotions compared to children who don't.

Although Gottman's book, *Raising the Emotionally Intelligent Child,* and website provide detailed information about the steps, here is a brief summary:

Accept and listen

Be accepting of your child's negative emotions. Listen to your child to figure out what's going on.

Label the emotion and validate

Help your child figure out what they are feeling, as in "You sound like you are angry and that's okay. That makes sense because you really want more screen time don't you?"

Address the poor behaviors and come up with better ones

"But it's not okay for you to scream like that. Take a deep breath and let's talk about it." Later, you can talk with your child about possible solutions to the situation. Maybe it's giving more cues that screen time will be over or something else. Be sure to have your child help come up with solutions.

Remember, children's brains are still developing and they are learning how to manage the range of emotions. As parents, we can help them through this process so they can grow into emotionally intelligent adults. Using mindfulness can also help.

Mindfulness

Mindfulness is a simple technique that can help families manage stress. According to mindfulness pioneer Jon Kabat-Zinn, "Mindfulness is awareness that arises through paying attention, on purpose, in the present moment, non-judgmentally."[10] Unfortunately, our mind isn't always our friend. Thoughts can go a mile a minute, making situations seem more dire than they are. Mindfulness helps us see our lives with more clarity and to make better decisions.

One key aspect of formal mindfulness training is to help people accept unpleasant feelings without reacting to them, avoiding them, or being self-critical. This in turn improves self-regulation of emotions and behavior. In recent years, adult mindfulness programs have been adapted for children by shortening the duration, simplifying the language, and adding age-appropriate activities. Preliminary research with children show mindfulness programs help to reduce stress, anxiety, and improve attention and executive function.[11]

One program adapted for kids is the Hawn Foundation's (created by Goldie Hawn) MindUp, a curriculum used to promote social-emotional learning in school. A key part of the curriculum is teaching mindfulness. Children learn how to pay attention to their breathing and participate in exercises that help them stay in the present moment. Brain scans with adults reveal that those who practice mindfulness have a more dense prefrontal cortex, the part of the brain that aids focus, reasoning, and decision-making. The same way physical exercise helps bodies get stronger, mindfulness helps the brain work more efficiently.[12]

Melli O'Brien is a mindfulness practitioner who runs the

site Mrs. Mindfulness. In her article "Six Ways To Teach Mindfulness To Children," she recommends keeping sessions short, about five minutes, and increasing as appropriate. The goal is to "keep introducing it and practicing in short bursts until the child becomes more accustomed," she said. "With regular practice, you'll find kids not only getting better at the techniques, but using them of their own accord."[13]

O'Brien recommends having kids sit and close their eyes paying attention to their breathing. Have them do this for five cycles of breathing in and out. When they are done, ask them if they noticed any thoughts coming up and just to let them go and repeat the breathing. Try other mindful activities periodically during eating, walking, and play. Always start with some simple breathing exercises. For eating, have them chew slowly and pay close attention to the taste and texture of the food. Walking might include paying attention to how the ground feels underneath their feet. During play, be aware of the textures of finger-paint or any other sensory activity. When kids get distracted (and they will!), encourage them to focus on their senses and what they're experiencing.

Mindfulness is yet another tool you can use to help your child deal effectively with daily stress.

Deal with Stress Effectively Summary

Teaching kids how to deal with stress effectively takes time, investigative work, and a mind shift in how we view children's behavior. Below is a review of the key points in this chapter. Don't forget to check the resources in the back of the book if you want to learn more.

1) Practice the trifecta of self-care, which includes good sleep, a balanced and nutritious diet, and regular physical activity. These three lifestyle factors make it easier for you and your child to self-regulate behavior and emotions. Look for ways to practice healthy routines together as a family.

2) Identify hidden stressors and stress behaviors. Hidden stressors include noise, clutter, life disturbances, too much screen time, not enough activity, poor diet, peer issues, school work, and overstimulation. Stress behaviors may include trouble paying attention, difficulty with simple tasks, acting crabby, frequent emotional outbursts, overeating, trouble sleeping, and defiant behaviors.

3) Improve self-regulation by lowering the stressors (when able) or managing them better. Teach kids what it feels like to be calm and alert versus agitated or lethargic. Look for ways to get back to that "calm and alert" feeling such as moving their body, music, art, or some other activity.

4) Become an emotion coach by helping kids manage difficult emotions by accepting them, listening, and labeling/validating their feelings. Address behaviors that aren't acceptable and help your child replace them with more appropriate behaviors.

5) Work mindfulness into the day. Take time to be mindful by sitting in silence, watching breathing, and stopping to be present during everyday activities. Incorporate deep breathing when stress runs high.

6) Practice your own self-regulation strategies, so you are better able to help your child do the same. Make self-regulation a priority for the entire family.

Next, making sure that through it all parent and child stay connected.

PRINCIPLE 8

CONNECT WITH YOUR KIDS

*"I define connection as the energy that exists between
people when they feel seen, heard, and valued; when they
can give and receive without judgment; and when they
derive sustenance and strength from the relationship."*
–Brené Brown

A
nne's son, adopted from China at age three, was
food obsessed when he came to live with her and
her husband. Although weight was never an issue, it
was clear to Anne and her husband that their son did not
have a healthy relationship with food. They tried to let him
eat as much as he wanted for over a year, while he binged
and purged the food through chronic diarrhea. They were
trying times, to put it mildly, but they had faith he'd
eventually get the message that food was plentiful. "Our
son was hungry when food was visible and until the last
crumb was gone, but would show no signs of hunger when

all food was eaten or out of sight," she said. "It clearly was not a matter of physical hunger."

After a year they stopped letting him eat as much as he wanted because they felt it wasn't working. Although things got better after they took back control, some food challenge would always rear its ugly head. At school he'd seek food classmates dropped on the floor or discarded in trash bins, for example, or pester his peers incessantly for their lunch and snack items.

Fast-forward to age nine and Anne was still searching for answers. It wasn't until she read a book that changed the way she viewed his behavior that things took a positive turn. For the first time, she empathized with her son and how hard it must be for him. Her understanding tone struck a chord with him, and their relationship improved. She realized that this tension with food was keeping her and her husband from truly connecting with their son, and that was only fueling his food fixation. Now, he comes to her for hugs more often and she understands that the missing piece was never about food, but connection.

Emerging research shows the quality of the relationship between parents and children impact the risk of eating problems and obesity.[1] That means families with stronger emotional bonds, better communication, and more positive experiences fare better than those with constant friction, poor communication, and low bonding. So while it's our last of the 8 Principles of a healthy relationship with food, when it comes to your family's health and well-being, it may just be the most important.

The Food Framework – Substituting Food for Connection

Shelly and Dan had two kids, Gavin and Emmy. Their son

was athletic with a slim build and their daughter was round and less drawn to sports. Both Dan and Shelly were very active and played sports growing up. They encouraged both their children to be active, but it was Emmy they thought would benefit the most. They also felt like they had to watch her food more because of her weight. Though they tried to not make it noticeable, she got less access to sweets and was discouraged from second helpings. They were strict with their kids because they wanted well-behaved children, so outbursts were not tolerated and kids were sent straight to their room.

Emmy wanted to please her parents, so she tried hard at sports but deep down felt she wasn't as good as her teammates. Yet she could see her parents eyes light up when she had a good game and their disappointment when she didn't, so when it was time to sign up she always said yes. Beginning to feel like she didn't measure up, she started to eat for comfort. She would sneak more cookies at family parties and at home when her parents weren't looking. When they found out, they punished her, and food became even more of a sticking point.

Emmy's parents thought helping Emmy was about food and exercise, but underneath it all she was feeling bad about herself for not living up to their expectations. Her relationship with food slowly changed as she used it to fill a void that was getting bigger by the day. This feeling of unworthiness – and disconnection from her parents – led Emmy to sneak-eat, followed by guilt and shame.

Authoritarian Parenting

We touched on feeding styles (permissive, controlling, and moderate) in Principles 1 and 2, but the concept is actually born from the more extensive literature on parenting styles. In the 1970s, psychologist Diana Baumrind identified two important characteristics of parenting: structure and warmth.[2] Authoritarian style parenting is high on structure and expectations but is low in warmth and responsiveness. This is unlike authoritative parenting that is high on structure and expectations but also high on warmth and responsiveness. One review looking at 20 years of research showed that kids of authoritative parents were less likely to become depressed and get involved with risky behaviors like substance abuse.[3]

A big part of the problem with authoritarian parenting is the lack of sensitive responses to children. This means children are less likely to develop a secure attachment with their parents, and may shy away from going to them when they are stressed or in need of help. Research suggests this can lead to unhealthy physiological responses to stress, poorer self-regulation, and a loss of connection between parent and child.[4]

Emmy's parents were good people who always told their daughter they loved her. But in their pursuit to raise kids to behave properly, they missed out on helping Emmy grow emotionally and, to her, their acceptance felt conditional. This drove an invisible wedge between Emmy and her parents when food became a problem they didn't understand. The more they tried to control the food part, the worse the problem got.

As discussed in Principle 6, the difference between guilt and shame are important in these cases. "I believe that guilt is adaptive and helpful – it's holding something we've done or failed to do up against our values and feeling psychological discomfort," said shame researcher Brené Brown on her website. "I define shame as the intensely painful feeling or experience of believing that we are flawed and therefore unworthy of love and belonging – something we've experienced, done, or failed to do makes us unworthy of connection."[5]

When kids fall short of their parents' standards – and get punished for it or don't have a way to express their feelings – they may assume they are bad, allowing shame to take root and grow. But giving up on authoritarian parenting doesn't mean giving up on limits or teaching kids appropriate behavior. It just means you do it in a way that they know there's a difference between *their behavior* being unacceptable and *them* being unacceptable. It is more effective and keeps you connected so your child feels worthy and actually learns the lesson at hand.

Looking for Connection

Anne, introduced at the beginning of the chapter, felt her son was addicted to food, something he learned early in life at the orphanage. It's typical in society to label such an addiction as a brain disease for which the only answer is abstinence and self-control. But Anne realized that years of trying to suppress her son's food desires wasn't a long-term solution. "It's the constraining of the food that's problematic," said Marc Lewis, PhD, introduced in Principle 4. "Conflict makes something emotionally charged and that makes it more salient." In other words, conflict is a sure-fire way to make something even more desirable.

In his book, *The Biology of Desire,* Lewis makes the case that addiction isn't a disease at all, but a well-learned, albeit extreme, habit. It's the experiences that get repeated most often, he explains, that actually change the structure and function of the brain. Intense desire is what boosts the rate of learning in addictive-like behaviors. But at the core of most addictions is some type of hole that needs filling as Lewis explains in his book:

In each addiction narrative, we can see an underlying

current of anxiety, anger, or fear of rejection, and an
unconscious collusion between the child and his or her
caregivers to accept the burden of adequacy. That
collusion is exhausting. It creates a kind of emotional
starvation. With most addictions, this starvation
rebounds into desperate and repeated attempts at self-
fulfillment. The highs we get from X are extreme antidotes
to inner emptiness.[6]

This can be further explained using what psychologists call self-determination theory, which states that every human has certain psychological needs. These include a feeling of competence (confidence in reaching goals), relatedness (feeling connected to family and friends) and autonomy (feeling in control of one's life). Satisfying these needs is an important part of growth and fulfillment.[7]

When these needs aren't met, people look for ways to compensate with what researchers call "need substitutes" or "compensatory behaviors." Need substitutes take the form of externally-based goals like getting attention for the way you look, having money, getting straight A's, or being popular. This is different from intrinsically-based goals that focus on personal growth, nurturing relationships, and building health. Striving for external goals makes everything look good on the outside, but inside is a desperate need for approval that is never sated. Compensatory behaviors, on the other hand, are attempts to escape from bad feelings resulting from not getting one's needs met and may include abusing alcohol, binging on food, or spending money. In other words, it distracts people from the fact that something is missing in their lives. As Lewis explains in his book, it increases their desire for whatever is filling the void.

Anne noticed that in every picture of her son in the orphanage, he had food in his hands. This compensatory behavior was learned very early in life as he was vying for attention in a house full of kids. It was this behavior that compromised the connection between her and her son. While we tend to associate difficult childhoods with more extreme cases like child abuse or poverty, there's a spectrum. "It's any emotional friction with some people more vulnerable due to their temperaments," said Lewis. "This is why shame doesn't work – it's a painful emotion and then you need more of the stuff to cover up the pain. It's the worst type of pain there is." Think about it. Someone is feeling disconnected to others and more shame from loved ones only magnifies this disconnection. Then they feel an even stronger desire to fill up the hole.

The good news is the brain is malleable and can change in a more positive direction. More positive habits can be learned and connection, acceptance, and communication is the key.

The Mindful Framework – Connecting and Communicating

Shelly and Dan could sense something wasn't right with their daughter. When all the constraints on food weren't helping, and they found her sneaking, they stepped back to get some perspective. First, they stopped restricting her more than her brother but maintained regular mealtimes and offered sweets a few times per week. Shelly started spending more time with Emmy and both her and Dan became more tolerant and empathetic of her outbursts, while staying firm on expected behavior.

As Emmy felt more comfortable with her mom, she opened up about how she felt she wasn't really good at sports. Together they decided she would try something different which included musical theater, as she always had a creative flare. Instead of structured sports, she decided to spend time outdoors to stay active. Emmy began to feel more connected to her parents and often went to her mom when she had difficulties in school, and her mom listened and supported her in coming up with solutions. Emmy's relationship with food gradually improved as she no longer needed it to feel better and was able to eat until satisfaction.

Instead of just high expectations, Shelly and Dan also became more accepting and sensitive to their daughter's feelings, even when they didn't agree with them. This helped Emmy develop a positive sense of self-worth because she felt accepted for who she was and no longer needed food in the same way.

Authoritative Parenting & Connection

A strong body of evidence suggests authoritative parenting produces the most positive childhood outcomes. Again, it's this mixture of structure and high expectations with warmth and sensitive responsiveness that leads to a secure attachment between parent and child. This secure attachment improves children's physiological response to stress, and results in a high quality relationship between parent and child.[4]

Parenting Styles Elements		
Parenting Style	*Structure/High Expectations*	*Warmth/Sensitive Responses*
Authoritative	↑	↑
Authoritarian	↑	↓
Permissive	↓	↑

This positive relationship impacts healthy habits, too. In one study, taking data from project EAT (Eating and Activity in Teens), family functioning – communication, closeness, problem solving, and level of behavioral support – was shown to fuel healthy habits. For teen girls, higher family functioning was linked to lower weights, less sedentary behavior, increased fruit and vegetable intake, and higher breakfast and family meals. For boys, higher family functioning was associated with more activity, less fast food consumption, and more family meals.[8]

Strong relationships are also protective in and of themselves. In his well-received TED Talk, Dr. Robert Waldinger revealed the surprising results of a 75-year Harvard study examining what makes people happy and healthy. The study has followed 724 men over 75 years with 60 men left and has evolved to include the men's children and wives. Every two years the study participants are interviewed, have blood drawn, and are asked to produce health records.[9] Waldinger began his talk citing a survey that shows how millennials overwhelmingly believe that getting rich and becoming famous are keys to happiness (remember those external goals?), which is in direct contradiction to the Harvard study results.

"The lessons aren't about wealth or fame or working harder and harder," Waldinger said. "The clearest message that we get from the 75-year study is this: *good relationships keep us happy and healthy, period.*" He explains that people who are more connected in their relationships are happier and physically healthier, while those who are disconnected and lonely experience shorter life spans with less happiness and overall health. But it's not just the number of friends a person has or being in any relationship that matters – it's the quality of those close relationships. "It turns out, living in conflict is bad for our health," he said. In fact, this 75-year study shows that people in the most satisfying relationships at age 50 ended up being the healthiest at age 80 and beyond.

Nurturing supportive relationships can be hard if you grew up in a home where this was not the norm. That's what happened with Allison (in the last principle) so she educated herself and started anew. No matter what has happened in the past, change is always possible with a new outlook. The resource section can give you the additional help you need to get started.

Wholehearted Parenting

Brené Brown's research on shame sheds light on how parents can work towards what she calls "wholehearted parenting." It's helping children be courageous and resilient with connection at the core, by focusing on these key points:[10]

Make your home a safe haven

Children are often beat up out in the real world. They need home to be a place of nourishment, not just in relation to food but love and comfort. It's important to remember that kids work hard to control their impulses all day at school, so they tend to let loose at home. Creating an atmosphere of acceptance, love, and belonging is key. Brown's research shows that resilient teens believe they are worthy of deep connection. It's a parent's job to instill this belief in their children and themselves.

Avoid using shame in parenting

Brown's research shows children who are what she calls "shame prone" are more likely to engage in risky behavior compared to those who are "guilt prone." The key is helping children see that it's their behavior that needs to change, or they made the wrong choice, but that *they* are still wonderful and loved. This can be achieved by staying calm when kids misbehave and explaining why the behavior is inappropriate. But if, instead, parents yell and punish excessively, kids may assume they are flawed as a person. As Brown said in her book *Daring Greatly:* "If we can share our story with someone who responds with empathy and understanding, shame can't survive."

Set boundaries

As discussed in Principle 1, healthy boundaries are how children practice their self-control muscle. Brown said kids are hardwired to push against limits, but having boundaries is what makes children feel secure and safe in the world. It also shows parents care enough to set limits instead of letting kids do whatever they want.

Connection and Communication Basics

Communicating effectively also makes a world of difference. In addition to emotion coaching mentioned in Principle 7, the following tips help you fight fair, communicate better, and stay calm when kids aren't:

Use active listening

Active listening is a technique many therapists use, and it starts with listening carefully and then repeating what you think you heard and labeling feelings (sad, angry, disappointed, etc.).[11] For example, if a child is upset that she is getting less attention than her sibling, you wouldn't deny her feelings by saying "of course you get the same attention, that's ridiculous." You would try to understand her stance and repeat it back in your own words, "So you are saying that you think your younger sister gets more attention from us because we cuddle her more, and that makes you sad. Is that right?" This helps because not only do kids feel heard, it opens both parent and child up to solutions instead of the typical blame-game fight that goes nowhere.

Use "I" statements

In the 1960s, Thomas Gordon developed the concept of "I" statements to focus on the speaker's feelings.[12] This language is less accusatory than the typical "you" statements and gets to the heart of the issue sooner. You might say, "It hurts my feelings when you complain about meals because I work hard to prepare them," for example, instead of, "You always complain and are so ungrateful for all my hard work." When someone feels blamed or are made out to be a bad person, they get defensive and stop listening. But when you make it about your feelings – instead of the other person's attributes – you can get your message across. This type of communication not only brings families closer, it's more likely to end in resolution and understanding.

Try not to jump in with advice

One of my biggest challenges has been giving my daughter advice while she was upset instead of listening and understanding. This tendency of mine only made her more upset and she felt like I didn't understand. But in my mind, I felt that I knew the answer and wanted to save the day! What I came to realize is she needed to figure things out for herself, and by giving her the answers, I was short-changing her emotional growth. Later, when she was calm, I could share stories with her and a bit of advice, but most of the advice came when she actually asked for it.

Spend one-on-one time with your child

According to research, spending time with your child is more about quality than quantity.[13] Make sure most days you spend time together engaging with each other. Turn off the phones, iPad, and TV so there are no distractions. Kids crave our time and attention, and just being with them helps them recognize their importance.

Practice Makes Connections

This last principle provides the tools you need to connect and communicate with your child. This can take practice, but it's worth it when you notice your child coming to you for help and you see how a strong familial connection – and communication – makes the whole family happier and healthier.

Connect with Your Kids Summary

Connecting with kids is often missed when parents problem-solve their child's less-than-healthy habits. Even if this doesn't appear to be an issue, promoting connection with your child is an investment that boosts everyone's health. Here's a quick summary of this chapter's main points:

1) Quality relationships between parent and child help protect kids from eating problems and addictive-like behaviors. Commit to raising the quality of your relationship with your child at each stage of their development.

2) Aim for an authoritative parenting style that is high on structure and expectations but also rich in acceptance

and responsiveness. That means you support and empathize with your child as he struggles to do the right thing, even when staying firm on limits.

3) Ask if your child's core need for connection is being met, and if not, is your child compensating in some unhealthy way? If so, is their problematic behavior making it difficult to connect with him or her? If the answer is yes, make connection your focus, not changing the behavior.

4) Create a home that feeds connection by developing a safe haven where kids can share their struggles without feeling shamed. When kids make mistakes, be sure they understand it was the behavior, not who they are as a person, that needs changing. When you get it wrong – like yelling or losing your cool – be sure to apologize. This shows kids you make mistakes, too, but try to remedy them.

5) Promote positive communication by active listening and using "I" statements to get your messages across. Spend one-on-one time with your child on a regular basis to keep communication and connection a priority.

You now have 8 Powerful Principles to revolutionize your child's relationship with food and raise a mindful eater. The next chapter summarizes these principles so you can refer to them when life gets messy, something it tends to do quite often.

PROBLEM SOLVE WITH
THE 8 PRINCIPLES

Now that you are done with the book, I hope you experience few bumps on your journey. But I realize some bumps are to be expected. And it's not the bumps so much but how they are viewed and handled that is important. Although each of the 8 Principles work to help you raise a mindful eater, they also help you find solutions when problems creep up.

What exactly is a problem? Typically, it's the sense that your child's eating is off. Usually it consists of either the *how much* of eating or the *what* (or sometimes, both). You may be concerned that your child is eating less or more food than you think is right for her, which may (or may not) cause changes to weight. Then there's the *what* of eating. A child may become fixated on goodies or fast food, asking for them all the time, or showing little interest in nutritious foods.

Below are key questions you can ask to find answers. Always start with Internal Approaches, and if the answer doesn't come up there, go down the line. When you get that "aha," you will feel confident where the problem lies, and what you can do to help. Review the principle in question and see the Resource page to get additional help.

Internal Approaches to Eating

Principles 1 and 2 are all about structuring meals, setting limits, paying attention, and eating based on internal cues of hunger and fullness. If you sense your child is eating too much or too little, ask yourself these key questions:

Principle 1

- Am I planning meals and snacks to provide a regular rhythm and variety of offerings?
- Is meal structure loosening up? Are food limits being enforced?
- Is my child taking over my job of feeding (the what, when, and where), contributing to his eating in the absence of hunger? Is too much grazing causing him not to eat at meals?
- Is it time to change the timing of meals (take away a snack, add a snack, or change the timing of a main meal)?

Principle 2

- Am I taking over my child's job (the how much and what is eaten), potentially disconnecting him from internal cues of hunger and fullness?
- Am I serving meals family style or in a way that helps my child get the amount of food he needs?
- Is my child paying attention while eating or is he distracted?

- Is my child tuned into hunger and fullness when eating? Am I referring to hunger and fullness cues when I ask if she wants more food or is done?

Balance Food for Nourishment and Enjoyment

Principles 3, 4 and 5 help you find lasting ways to make nutrition rewarding, sweets less desirable, and eating well a pleasurable experience. If you find your child is fixated on goodies or shows little interest in a variety of food, these questions will help you get to the bottom of it:

Principle 3

- Why is my child so focused on goodies? Does she feel restricted? Are there too many food rewards?
- Where is my child in his development? Is this playing a role in his cravings? How are my feeding practices helping or harming?
- Is my child getting too much exposure to goodies compared to other foods?
- Is our flexible goodies policy still working? Is it time to increase/decrease or change something?

Principle 4

- Am I pushing nutritious food too much? Are nutrition messages positive, relating back to the interests of my child?
- Does my child have opportunities to experiment and learn about a variety of food?
- Is my child being exposed to a variety of food from all the food groups at meals and snacks?

- Are the nutrition messages I'm sending developmentally appropriate?

Principle 5

- Are meals enjoyable or a drag for my child? If it's a drag, how may it be contributing to her feelings about food?
- Are there regular opportunities for my child to help with meals?
- Do we have food rituals that get my child interested in meals? Do we show gratitude for food on a regular basis?

Body Appreciation and Self-care

Principles 6 and 7 give you the tools to teach your child how to appreciate her body, to develop a positive body image, and to learn the art of self-care. If you find your child eating erratically, it may be she is trying to change her body with food. Here are the questions to ask to see if you need to focus on body appreciation:

Principle 6

- Where is my child on the eating behavior spectrum? A normal eater, disordered eater, or even signs of an eating disorder?
- Do I understand my child's growth? Is it on track or are there deviations? What has changed to bring deviations in growth?
- Is my child comparing herself to her peers' bodies? What impact may this be having on her own thoughts about her body?

- What else is happening at school? Could there be teasing or friends' influence?
- If she doesn't like her body, does she feel shame? Is this related to her eating more at times (emotional eating)? Does my child understand the three lessons of a positive body image? Is the self-esteem culture affecting her or is she able to utilize self-compassion?

Principle 7

- Is my child practicing (with my support) the trifecta of self-care? Is he getting enough sleep, eating balanced meals, and getting physical activity on a regular basis? Does he understand how this relates to having a strong and healthy body?

Mental and Emotional Happiness

Principles 7 and 8 help you teach your child the art of self- and emotional regulation, identifying and dealing with stressors, and making connection between parent and child a priority. If you feel you have done everything and still can't find answers to changes in eating in either the how much or what, it may lie in the emotion and stress realm.*Principle 7*

- Are there hidden stressors affecting my child's ability to self-regulate? Are these misbehaviors or stress behaviors?
- Does my child know how to manage the stressor? Does she know how to get back to calm?
- Is my child having trouble processing difficult emotions? Have I been there to coach her on emotions?

- Am I practicing and modeling self-regulation skills? What can I do to be a better role model?

Principle 8

- Do I feel connected to my child? Could I improve upon the quality of our relationship? Are problems with food getting in the way of this connection?
- Am I (and my partner) practicing authoritative parenting: structure and limits with warmth and sensitive responses? Does my child feel like she can come to me with her problems?
- If my child doesn't feel connected or good about himself, is he compensating with food? Or is he hyper-focused on other areas (grades, popularity, etc.) as a need substitute?
- Am I practicing helpful communication skills like active listening and "I" statements to get my message across?
- Are both my partner and I spending quality time with my child on a regular basis?

When you master all of the 8 Principles – and use them to problem-solve – it will feel like you have a secret. I wrote this book to let the secret out once and for all. Every parent should know there is a different – and better – way to raise children around food. If you find you are having trouble problem-solving, or feel this book does not address an important issue, feel free contact me by going to my website MaryannJacobsen.com. Your feedback will help make future editions of *How to Raise a Mindful Eater* even better.

May your family reap the benefits of a happy and healthy relationship with food now and in the years to come.

RESOURCES

Internal Approaches to Eating

- *Intuitive Eating: A Revolutionary Program That Works* by Evelyn Tribole and Elsye Resch
- *Eat What You Love, Love What You Eat* by Michelle May
- The Center for Mindful Eating http://thecenterformindfuleating.org/
- Megrette Fletcher website https://mindfuleatingforkids.wordpress.com/ and book *Discover Mindful Eating for Kids* by Megrette Fletcher
- Ellyn Satter Institute http://www.ellynsatterinstitute.org/ and books by Ellyn Satter including *Your Child's Weight, Helping Without Harming*
- Geneen Roth's website https://geneenroth.com/ and books including *Women, Food and God* (focused on emotional eating)
- Private Facebook Page for parents struggling with their child's food obsession: send friend request to Bonnie Appetites

- Super Healthy Kids Meal Planning System https://www.superhealthykids.com/meal-plan-memberships/
- Six O'Clock Scramble Meal Planning Tool http://www.thescramble.com/
- *The Family Dinner Solution: How to Create a Rotation of Dinner Meals Your Family Will Love* by Maryann Jacobsen

Balance Food for Nourishment and Enjoyment

- *Fearless Feeding: How to Raise Healthy Eaters from High Chair to High School* by Jill Castle and Maryann Jacobsen
- *How to Teach Nutrition to Kids* by Connie Evers
- *Finding Your Way to Change: How the Power of Motivational Interviewing Can Reveal What You Want and Help You Get There* by Allan Zuckoff
- *The Snactivist's Handbook: How to Change the Junk Food Snack Culture at School, in Sports, and Camp —and Raise Healthier Snackers at Home* by Sally Kuzemchak http://www.realmomnutrition.com/snacktivists-handbook/
- The Kids Healthy Weight Project by Jill Castle (online course) http://jillcastle.com/courses/

Body Appreciation and Self Care

- *Body Respect: What Conventional Health Books Get Wrong, Leave Out, and Just Plain Fail to Understand About Weight* by Linda Bacon
- Kathy Kater's Healthy Bodies Curriculum http://bodyimagehealth.org/healthy-bodies-curriculum/ and *Healthy Bodies: Teaching Kids What They Need to Know: A Comprehensive Curriculum to*

Address Body Image, Eating, Fitness and Weight Concerns in Today's Challenging Environment (Volume 3)
- *Sexualulized Media Messages and Our Children: Teaching Kids to Be Smart Critics and Consumers* by Jennifer Shewmaker
- *No Sweat: How the Science of Motivation Can Bring You a Lifetime of Fitness* by Michelle Segar
- Health at Every Size http://haescommunity.com/
- Ways for Parents to Combat Weight Bias by The Rudd Center for Food Policy and Obesity http://www.uconnruddcenter.org/resources/upload/docs/what/bias/parents/Parents-WaystoCombatWeightBias.pdf
- Dr. Stuart Shanker Merhit Center https://self-reg.ca/about-us-4/dr-stuart-shanker/ and book *Self Reg: How to Help Your Child (and You) Break the Stress Cycle and Successfully Engage with Life*

Mental and Emotional Happiness
- Laura Markham's website Aha Parenting http://www.ahaparenting.com/ and book *Peaceful Parent, Happy Child*
- The Gottman Institute site https://www.gottman.com/ and book by John Gottman: *Raising an Emotionally Intelligent Child*
- *How to Talk so Kids Will Listen & Listen so Kids Will Talk* by Adele Faber and Elaine Mazlish
- Thomas Gordon Parent Effectiveness Training (P.E.T.) http://www.gordontraining.com/parent-programs/parent-effectiveness-training-p-e-t/
- Amy McCready's website and books https://www.positiveparentingsolutions.com/

- *Self-Compassion: The Proven Power of Being Kind to Yourself* by Kristen Neff
- Mrs. Mindfulness website, classes, and retreats http://mrsmindfulness.com/
- The Hawn Foundation Mind Up https://mindup.org/
- Jon Kabat-Zinn mindfulness books https://www.amazon.com/Jon-Kabat-Zinn/e/B000AQ12GA
- Tara Brach website, guided meditations, and books https://www.tarabrach.com/
- *The Mayo Clinic Guide to Stress-Free Living* by Amit Sood.
- Brené Brown website and books http://brenebrown.com/

Accelerated Growth/Weight Issues
- Find a dietitian at Eatright.org/find-an-expert under pediatric obesity/weight management
- Shapedown: Weight Management for Children and Adolescents http://www.shapedown.com/

Books for Kids
- *Amanda's Big Dream* by Judith Matz and Elizabeth Patch
- *What Does Your Tummy Say?* by Maryann Jacobsen
- *When you Worry too Much* by Dawn Heubner and Bonnie Matthews

New Thinking/Approaches to Addiction
- *The Biology of Desire: Why Addiction is Not a Disease* by Marc Lewis
- *The Unbroken Brain: A Revolutionary New Way of Understanding Addiction* by Maria Svalavitz

ABOUT THE AUTHOR

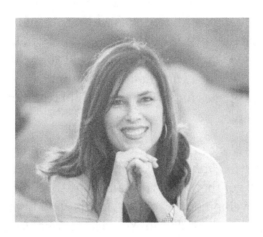

Maryann Jacobsen is a registered dietitian, independent author, and speaker. She is founding editor of Raise Healthy Eaters (now MaryannJacobsen.com) and runs The Healthy Family Podcast. Maryann's books, blog, and podcast aim to revolutionize the health of families through improving their relationship with food. Her writing has appeared in the New York Times, Los Angeles Times, Mindbodygreen, and She Knows. She has been quoted in various publications including *Parents, Scholastic Parent & Child* and *American Profile* and has been featured on *Good Morning America.* Find out more at MaryannJacobsen.com.

Other titles by Maryann Jacobsen include:

The Family Dinner Solution: How to Create a Rotation of Dinner Meals Your Family Will Love: In a step-by-step format, you will learn how to create a core rotation of dinner meals that will satisfy even your pickiest family members. The result? You'll never, ever have to worry about what to cook for dinner again!

From Picky to Powerful: The Mindset, Strategies and Know-How You Need to Empower Your Picky Eater: By explaining the scientific reasons why most children become picky in the first place – and the importance of individual differences — you'll come to understand your child's eating behaviors. *From Picky to Powerful* outlines specific and effective strategies for feeding your child based on the latest research.

Fearless Feeding: How to Raise Healthy Eaters From High Chair to High School: Considered the bible of feeding kids, you'll get the What, How and Why of feeding at each stage of development — infancy, toddlerhood, school age, adolescence and adulthood. You'll learn what to expect in terms of growth, child development (the why of eating) and how to meet nutritional needs.

What Does Your Tummy Say? is a children's story that highlights the importance of tuning into hunger and fullness. It can serve as a conversation starter for families to share experiences and challenges, and learn about healthy ways to relate to food.

Sign up for Maryann's email list and get her FREE e-book, *10 Things Never to Say to Your Child About Food.* Go to MaryannJacobsen.com/list.

NOTES

Introduction

1) Tavernise, Sabrina. "Obesity Rises Despite All Efforts to Fight It, US Officials Say." New York Times. November 12, 15. Accessed July 7, 16. http://www.nytimes.com/2015/11/12/health/obesity-rises-despite-all-efforts-to-fight-it-us-health-officials-say.html.

2) Lowe, Michael R., Sapna D. Doshi, Shawn N. Katterman, and Emily H. Feig. "Dieting and Restrained Eating as Prospective Predictors of Weight Gain." *Frontiers in Psychology*, 4 (2013). doi:10.3389/fpsyg.2013.00577.

3) US Department of Health and Human Services; US Department of Agriculture. *2015-2020 Dietary Guidelines for Americans*. 8th ed. Washington, DC: US Dept. of Health and Human Services; December 2015. http://www.health.gov/DietaryGuidelines. Accessed March 14, 2016.

4) Bellisle, France. "Meals and Snacking, Diet Quality and Energy Balance." *Physiology & Behavior,* 134 (July 2014): 38–43. doi:10.1016/j.physbeh.2014.03.010.

5) Ahmad, Qazi Iqbal, Charoo Bashir Ahmad, and Sheikh Mushtaq Ahmad. "Childhood Obesity." *Indian Journal of Endocrinology & Metabolism,* 14, no. 1 (2010).

6) Office of The Surgeon General. *A Call To Action To Prevent and Decrease Overweight and Obesity.* Rockville, MD: U.S. Dept. of Health and Human Services, Public Health Service, 2001. http://www.cdc.gov/nccdphp/dnpa/pdf/calltoaction.pdf.

7) Letsmove. "America's Move to Raise A Healthier Generation of Kids." Accessed October 12, 2016. http://www.letsmove.gov/about.

8) Saguy, Abigail C. and Rene Almeling. "Fat in the Fire? Science, the News Media, and the 'Obesity Epidemic' 2." *Sociological Forum,* 23, no. 1 (October 26, 2007): 53–83. doi:10.1111/j.1600-0838.2004.00399.x-ii.

9) Zander, Rosamund Stone and Benjamin Zander. *The Art of Possibility: Transforming Professional and Personal Life.* Reprint Edition. New York, New York: Penguin Books, 2002.

Challenging the Old Way

1) Tyler, David B. "The Biology of Human Starvation. Two Volumes. Ancel Keys Josef Brozek Austin Henschel Olaf Mickelsen Henry Longstreet Taylor Ernst Simonson Angie Sturgeon Skinner Samuel M. Wells." *The Quarterly Review of Biology,* 26, no. 1 (March 1951): 88–89. doi:10.1086/397995.

2) Kalm, Leah M., and Richard D. Semba. "They Starved So That Others Be Better Fed: Remembering Ancel Keys and the Minnesota Experiment." *The Journal of Nutrition,* 135, no. 6 (June 1, 2005): 1347-352.

3) Fisher, Jennifer O., and Leann L. Birch. "Restricting Access to Palatable Foods Affects Children's Behavioral Response, Food Selection, and Intake." *American Journal of Clinical Nutrition,* 69, no. 6 (June 1999): 1264-272.

4) Fisher, Jennifer O., and Leann L. Birch. "Eating in the Absence of Hunger and Overweight in Girls from 5 to 7 Y of Age." *American Journal of Clinical Nutrition,* 76, no. 1 (July 2002): 226-31.

5) Rollins, Brandi Y., Eric Loken, Jennifer S. Savage, and Leann L. Birch. "Effects of Restriction on Children's Intake Differ by Child Temperament, Food Reinforcement, and Parent's Chronic Use of Restriction." *Appetite,* 73 (2014): 31-39. doi:10.1016/j.appet.2013.10.005.

6) Scaqlioni, S., C. Arrizza, F. Vecchi, and S. Tedeschi. "Determinants of Children's Eating Behavior." *American Journal of Clinical Nutrition*, Supplement, 94, no. 6 (December 2011): 2006S-2011S. doi:10.3945/ajcn.110.001685.

7) Birch, LL, JO Fisher, and KK Davison. "Learning to Overeat: Maternal Use of Restrictive Feeding Practices Promotes Girls' Eating in the Absence of Hunger." *The American Journal of Clinical Nutrition,* 78, no. 2 (July 30, 2003): 215–20.

8) Golden, N. H., M. Schneider, and C. Wood. "Preventing Obesity and Eating Disorders in Adolescents," *Pediatrics,* 138, no. 3 (August 22, 2016): e20161649– e20161649. doi:10.1542/peds.2016-1649.

9) Pietiläinen, K H, S E Saarni, J Kaprio, and A Rissanen. "Does Dieting Make You Fat? A Twin Study." *International Journal of Obesity,* 36, no. 3 (August 9, 2011): 456–64. doi:10.1038/ijo.2011.160.

10) French, S.A., L.H. Epstein, R.W. Jeffery, J.E. Blundell, and J Wardle. "Eating Behavior Dimensions.

Associations with Energy Intake and Body Weight. A Review." *Appetite*, 59, no. 2 (2012): 541–549. doi: 10.1016/j.appet.2012.07.001.

11) Müller, M. J. and A. Bosy-Westphal. "Adaptive Thermogenesis with Weight Loss in Humans." *Obesity*, 21, no. 2 (February 2013): 218–28. doi:10.1002/oby.20027.

12) Fothergill, Erin, Juen Guo, Lilian Howard, Jennifer C. Kerns, Nicolas D. Knuth, Robert Brychta, Kong Y. Chen, et al. "Persistent Metabolic Adaptation 6 Years After 'The Biggest Loser' Competition." *Obesity*, 24, no. 8 (May 2, 2016): 1612–19. doi:10.1002/oby.21538.

13) Martin, Corby K., Leonie K. Heilbronn, Lilian de Jonge, James P. DeLany, Julia Volaufova, Stephen D. Anton, Leanne M. Redman, Steven R. Smith, and Eric Ravussin. "Effect of Calorie Restriction on Resting Metabolic Rate and Spontaneous Physical Activity." *Obesity*, 15, no. 12 (December 2007): 2964–73. doi:10.1038/oby.2007.354.

14) Dulloo, A. G., J. Jacquet, J. P. Montani, and Y. Schutz. "How Dieting Makes the Lean Fatter: From a Perspective of Body Composition Autoregulation Through Adipostats and Proteinstats Awaiting Discovery." *Obesity Reviews*, 16 (January 22, 2015): 25–35. doi:10.1111/obr.12253.

15) American Psychiatric Association. *Feeding and Eating Disorders*. n.p., 2013. https://www.appi.org/feeding_and_eating_disorders.

16) H. Ziauddeen and P. C. Fletcher. "Is Food Addiction a Valid and Useful Concept?" *Obesity Reviews*, 14, no. 1 (October 12, 2012): 19–28. doi:10.1111/j.1467-789x.2012.01046.x.

17) McDermottMedically, Annette. "Is Cognitive Behavioral Therapy (CBT) an Effective Treatment for Binge Eating Disorder?" 2005. Accessed October 7,

2016. http://www.healthline.com/health/eating-disorders/cbt-for-binge-eating-disorder#2.

18) Hardman, C.A., P.J. Rogers, R. Dallas, J. Scott, H.K. Ruddock, and E. Robinson. "'Food Addiction is Real'". The Effects of Exposure to This Message on Self-Diagnosed Food Addiction and Eating Behaviour." *Appetite*, 91, (2015): 179–184. doi: 10.1016/j.appet.2015.04.052

19) Holohan, Meghan. *Mom Angry After School Sends Athletic 11-Year-Old Home with "fat letter."* (TODAY), October 8, 2013. Accessed November 10, 2016. http://www.today.com/parents/mom-angry-after-school-sends-athletic-11-year-old-home-8C11356010.

20) Flegal, Katherine M., Brian K. Kit, Heather Orpana, and Barry I. Graubard. "Association of All-Cause Mortality with Overweight and Obesity Using Standard Body Mass Index Categories." *JAMA,* 309, no. 1 (January 2, 2013): 71. doi:10.1001/jama.2012.113905.

21) Bunch, Jared T. "The Obesity Paradox: What Does Weight Have to Do with Longevity?" April 30, 2014. Accessed October 7, 2016. http://www.everydayhealth.com/columns/jared-bunch-rhythm-of-life/obesity-paradox-weight-longevity/.

22) Ogden, Cynthia L., Margaret D. Carroll, Brian K. Kit, and Katherine M. Flegal. "Prevalence of Childhood and Adult Obesity in the United States, 2011-2012." *JAMA,* 311, no. 8 (February 26, 2014): 806. doi:10.1001/jama.2014.732.

23) Roberson, Lara L, Ehimen C Aneni, Wasim Maziak, Arthur Agatston, Theodore Feldman, Maribeth Rouseff, Thinh Tran, et al. "Beyond BMI: The 'Metabolically Healthy Obese' Phenotype & Its Association with Clinical/Subclinical Cardiovascular Disease and All-Cause Mortality — a Systematic

Review." *BMC Public Health,* 14, no. 1 (January 8, 2014). doi:10.1186/1471-2458-14-14.

24) Bacon, Linda and Lucy Aphramor. "Weight Science: Evaluating the Evidence for a Paradigm Shift." *Nutrition Journal,* 10, no. 1 (2011): 9. doi:10.1186/1475-2891-10-9.

25) Cao, Sissi, Rahim Moineddin, Marcelo L Urquia, Fahad Razak, and Joel G Ray. "J-Shapedness: An Often Missed, Often Miscalculated Relation: The Example of Weight and Mortality." *Journal of Epidemiology and Community Health,* 68, no. 7 (March 28, 2014): 683–90. doi:10.1136/jech-2013-203439.

26) Mozes, Alan. *Underweight Even Deadlier Than Overweight, Study Says.* (HealthDay), March 28, 2014. Accessed November 10, 2016. https://consumer.healthday.com/senior-citizen-information-31/misc-death-and-dying-news-172/underweight-even-deadlier-than-overweight-study-says-686240.html.

27) Kaiser, K. A., A. W. Brown, M. M. Bohan Brown, J. M. Shikany, R. D. Mattes, and D. B. Allison. "Increased Fruit and Vegetable Intake Has No Discernible Effect on Weight Loss: A Systematic Review and Meta-Analysis." *American Journal of Clinical Nutrition,* 100, no. 2 (June 25, 2014): 567–76. doi:10.3945/ajcn.114.090548.

28) Tanofsky-Kraff, Marian, Ann Haynos, Lisa Kotler, Susan Yanovski, and Jack Yanovski. "Laboratory-Based Studies of Eating Among Children and Adolescents." *Current Nutrition & Food Science,* 3, no. 1 (February 1, 2007): 55–74. doi:10.2174/1573401310703010055.

29) CDC. "Short Sleep Duration Among Workers — United States, 2010." April 27, 2012. Accessed November 8, 2016.

https://www.cdc.gov/mmwr/preview/mmwrhtml/mm
6116a2.htm.

30) Owens, J. "Insufficient Sleep in Adolescents and Young
Adults: An Update on Causes and Consequences."
Pediatrics, 134, no. 3 (August 25, 2014): e921–32.
doi:10.1542/peds.2014-1696.

31) Chaput, Jean-Philippe. "Sleep Patterns, Diet Quality
and Energy Balance." *Physiology & Behavior,* 134 (July
2014): 86–91. doi:10.1016/j.physbeh.2013.09.006.

32) The American Institute of Stress. "FAQ's." August 29,
2011. Accessed November 8, 2016.
http://www.stress.org/about/faqs/.

33) Sinha, Rajita and Ania M. Jastreboff. "Stress as a
Common Risk Factor for Obesity and Addiction."
Biological Psychiatry, 73, no. 9 (May 2013): 827–35.
doi:10.1016/j.biopsych.2013.01.032.

34) Harvard School of Public Health. "Exercise Can Help
Control Weight." October 21, 2012. Accessed November
8, 2016. https://www.hsph.harvard.edu/obesity-
prevention-source/obesity-causes/physical-activity-
and-obesity/.

35) Jayawardene, Wasantha P., Mohammad R. Torabi, and
David K. Lohrmann. "Exercise in Young Adulthood
with Simultaneous and Future Changes in Fruit and
Vegetable Intake." *Journal of the American College of
Nutrition,* 35, no. 1 (August 7, 2015): 59–67.
doi:10.1080/07315724.2015.1022268.

36) Mintel Group Ltd. *A Snacking Nation: 94% of
Americans Snack Daily.* 2016. Accessed November 8,
2016. http://www.mintel.com/press-centre/food-and-
drink/a-snacking-nation-94-of-americans-snack-daily.

37) American Psychologic Association. "Stress and Eating."
2013. Accessed November 8, 2016.
http://www.apa.org/news/press/releases/stress/2013/
eating.aspx.

38) Robinson, E., P. Aveyard, A. Daley, K. Jolly, A. Lewis, D. Lycett, and S. Higgs. "Eating Attentively: A Systematic Review and Meta-Analysis of the Effect of Food Intake Memory and Awareness on Eating." *American Journal of Clinical Nutrition,* 97, no. 4 (February 27, 2013): 728–42. doi:10.3945/ajcn.112.045245.

39) Calorie Control Council. "Survey: Most Americans Are Weight Conscious." April 27, 2011. Accessed November 8, 2016. http://caloriecontrol.org/survey-most-americans-are-weight-conscious/.

40) Neumark-Sztainer, Dianne, Melanie Wall, Nicole I. Larson, Marla E. Eisenberg, and Katie Loth. "Dieting and Disordered Eating Behaviors from Adolescence to Young Adulthood: Findings from a 10-Year Longitudinal Study." *Journal of the American Dietetic Association,* 111, no. 7 (July 2011): 1004–11. doi:10.1016/j.jada.2011.04.012.

41) Evelyn Tribole and Elyse Resch. *Intuitive Eating: A Revolutionary Program That Works.* 3rd edition. New York, New York: Saint Martin's Griffin, 2012.

42) Tribole, Evelyn and Elyse Resch. What Is Intuitive Eating?" Accessed October 30, 2016. http://www.intuitiveeating.com/content/what-intuitive-eating.

43) Tylka, Tracy L. and Ashley M. Kroon Van Diest. "The Intuitive Eating Scale–2: Item Refinement and Psychometric Evaluation with College Women and Men." *Journal of Counseling Psychology,* 60, no. 1 (2013): 137–53. doi:10.1037/a0030893.

44) Tribole, Evelyn and Elyse Resch. "Intuitive Eating Studies." 2016. Accessed October 7, 2016. http://intuitiveeating.com/content/resources.

45) Denny, Kara N., Katie Loth, Marla E. Eisenberg, and Dianne Neumark-Sztainer. "Intuitive Eating in Young

Adults. Who Is Doing It, and How Is It Related to Disordered Eating Behaviors?" *Appetite,* 60 (January 2013): 13–19. doi:10.1016/j.appet.2012.09.029.

46) O'Reilly, G. A., L. Cook, D. Spruijt-Metz, and D. S. Black. "Mindfulness-Based Interventions for Obesity-Related Eating Behaviours: A Literature Review." *Obesity Reviews,* 15, no. 6 (March 18, 2014): 453–61. doi:10.1111/obr.12156.
47) Satter, Ellyn. "Eating Competence: Definition and Evidence for the Satter Eating Competence Model." *Journal of Nutrition Education and Behavior,* 39, no. 5 (2007): S142–53. Accessed October 7, 2016. doi:10.1016/j.jneb.2007.01.006. http://ellynsatterinstitute.org/cms-assets/documents/101150-596171.ecdefandev.pdf.

Principle 1

1) Shloim, Netalie, Lisa R. Edelson, Nathalie Martin, and Marion M. Hetherington. "Parenting Styles, Feeding Styles, Feeding Practices, and Weight Status in 4–12-Year-Old Children: A Systematic Review of the Literature." *Frontiers in Psychology,* 6 (December 14, 2015). doi:10.3389/fpsyg.2015.01849.
2) Musher-Eizenman, Dara R., Jenna M. Marx, and Maija B. Taylor. "It's Always Snack Time: An Investigation of Event Scripts in Young Children." *Appetite,* 85 (February 2015): 66–69. doi:10.1016/j.appet.2014.11.013.
3) Piernas, C. and B. M. Popkin. "Trends in Snacking Among U.S. Children." *Health Affairs,* 29, no. 3 (March 1, 2010): 398–404. doi:10.1377/hlthaff.2009.0666.
4) Isacco, L., N. Lazaar, S. Ratel, D. Thivel, J. Aucouturier, E. Doré, M. Meyer, and P. Duché. "The Impact of

Eating Habits on Anthropometric Characteristics in French Primary School Children." *Child Care, Health and Development,* 36, no. 6 (July 14, 2010): 835–42. doi:10.1111/j.1365-2214.2010.01113.x.

5) Satter, Ellyn. "Division of Responsibility in Feeding." 2016. Accessed October 7, 2016. http://ellynsatterinstitute.org/dor/divisionofresponsib ilityinfeeding.php.

6) Rollins, B. Y., J. S. Savage, J. O. Fisher, and L. L. Birch. "Alternatives to Restrictive Feeding Practices to Promote Self-Regulation in Childhood: A Developmental Perspective." *Pediatric Obesity,* 11, no. 5 (September 25, 2015): 326–32. doi:10.1111/ijpo.12071.

7) Markham, Laura. "Why Empathic Limits Help Kids Develop Self Control." 2016. Accessed October 7, 2016. http://www.ahaparenting.com/blog/The_Secret_of_R aising_a_Self-Disciplined_Child.

8) Laska, Melissa N, Mary O Hearst, Katherine Lust, Leslie A Lytle, and Mary Story. "How We Eat What We Eat: Identifying Meal Routines and Practices Most Strongly Associated with Healthy and Unhealthy Dietary Factors Among Young Adults." *Public Health Nutrition,* 18, no. 12 (December 2, 2014): 2135–45. doi:10.1017/s1368980014002717.

9) AAP Committee on Nutrition and Ronald E. Kleinman MD FAAP. *Pediatric Nutrition Handbook.* 6th edition. American Academy of Pediatrics, 2008.

10) Castle, Jill and Maryann Jacobsen. *Fearless Feeding: How to Raise Healthy Eaters from High Chair to High School.* San Francisco: Jossey-Bass, 2013.

Principle 2

1) Orrell-Valente, Joan K., Laura G. Hill, Whitney A. Brechwald, Kenneth A. Dodge, Gregory S. Pettit, and John E. Bates. "'Just three more bites': An Observational Analysis of Parents' Socialization of Children's Eating at Mealtime." *Appetite,* 48, no. 1 (January 2007): 37–45. doi:10.1016/j.appet.2006.06.006.

2) Loth, K. A., R. F. MacLehose, J. A. Fulkerson, S. Crow, and D. Neumark-Sztainer. "Food-Related Parenting Practices and Adolescent Weight Status: A Population-Based Study." *Pediatrics,* 131, no. 5 (April 22, 2013): e1443–e1450. doi:10.1542/peds.2012-3073.

3) Savage, Jennifer S., Jennifer Orlet Fisher, and Leann L. Birch. "Parental Influence on Eating Behavior: Conception to Adolescence." *The Journal of Law, Medicine & Ethics,* 35, no. 1 (March 2007): 22–34. doi:10.1111/j.1748-720x.2007.00111.x

4) Ellis, Jordan M., Amy T. Galloway, Rose Mary Webb, Denise M. Martz, and Claire V. Farrow. "Recollections of Pressure to Eat During Childhood, but Not Picky Eating, Predict Young Adult Eating Behavior." *Appetite,* 97 (February 2016): 58–63. doi:10.1016/j.appet.2015.11.020.

5) Farrow, C. V., E. Haycraft, and J. M. Blissett. "Teaching Our Children When to Eat: How Parental Feeding Practices Inform the Development of Emotional Eating--a Longitudinal Experimental Design." *American Journal of Clinical Nutrition* 101, no. 5 (March 18, 2015): 908–13. doi:10.3945/ajcn.114.103713.

6) Dockendorff, Sally A., Trent A. Petrie, Christy A. Greenleaf, and Scott Martin. "Intuitive Eating Scale: An

Examination Among Early Adolescents." *Journal of Counseling Psychology*, 59, no. 4 (2012): 604–11. doi:10.1037/a0029962.

7) Higgs, Suzanne and Jessica E. Donohoe. "Focusing on Food During Lunch Enhances Lunch Memory and Decreases Later Snack Intake." *Appetite*, 57, no. 1 (August 2011): 202–6. doi:10.1016/j.appet.2011.04.016.

8) Robinson, E., P. Aveyard, A. Daley, K. Jolly, A. Lewis, D. Lycette and S. Higgs. "Eating Attentively: A Systematic Review and Meta-Analysis of the Effect of Food Intake Memory and Awareness on Eating." *American Journal of Clinical Nutrition*, 97, no. 4 (February 27, 2013): 728–42. doi:10.3945/ajcn.112.045245.

9) Johnson, S. L. "Improving Preschoolers' Self-Regulation of Energy Intake." *Pediatrics*, 106, no. 6 (December 1, 2000): 1429–35. doi:10.1542/peds.106.6.1429.

10) Ramsay, Samantha A., Laurel J. Branen, Janice Fletcher, Elizabeth Price, Susan L. Johnson, and Madeleine Sigman-Grant. "'Are you done?' Child Care Providers' Verbal Communication at Mealtimes That Reinforce or Hinder Children's Internal Cues of Hunger and Satiation." *Journal of Nutrition Education and Behavior*, 42, no. 4 (July 2010): 265–70. doi:10.1016/j.jneb.2009.07.002.

11) Fletcher, Margaret. Discover Mindful Eating for Kids. Shelly Skills, 2015.

12) Stockman, J. A. "Risk Factors for Childhood Overweight: A Prospective Study from Birth to 9.5 Years." *Yearbook of Pediatrics*, 2006 (January 2006): 419–20. doi:10.1016/s0084-3954(07)70248-8.

13) Savage, Jennifer S., Leann L. Birch, Michele Marini, Stephanie Anzman-Frasca, and Ian M. Paul. "Effect of

the INSIGHT Responsive Parenting Intervention on Rapid Infant Weight Gain and Overweight Status at Age 1 Year." *JAMA Pediatrics,* 170, no. 8 (August 1, 2016): 742. doi:10.1001/jamapediatrics.2016.0445.

14) Indivero, Victoria M. "Intervention Reduces Rates of Overweight Tots by Half | Penn State University." October 30, 2016. Accessed October 30, 2016. http://news.psu.edu/story/413513/2016/06/06/resear ch/intervention-reduces-rates-overweight-tots-half.

Principle 3

1) Braet, C., G. O'Malley, D. Weghuber, A. Vania, E. Edhardt, P. Nowika, A. Mazur, M. L. Frelut, and E. Ardelt-Gattinger. *The Assessment of Eating Behaviour in Children Who Are Obese: A Psychological Approach. A Position Paper from the European Childhood Obesity Group.* Report no. 3. The European Child Obesity Group. Vol. 7. *Obesity Facts,* 2014. 153-64. Accessed October 9, 2016. http://www.karger.com/Article/FullText/362391.

2) Lu, Ji, Suhong Xiong, Narendra Arora, and Laurette Dubé. "Using Food as Reinforcer to Shape Children's Non-Food Behavior: The Adverse Nutritional Effect Doubly Moderated by Reward Sensitivity and Gender." *Eating Behaviors,* 19 (December 2015): 94–97. doi:10.1016/j.eatbeh.2015.07.003.

3) Puhl, Rebecca M and Marlene B Schwartz. "If You Are Good You Can Have a Cookie: How Memories of Childhood Food Rules Link to Adult Eating Behaviors." *Eating Behaviors,* 4, no. 3 (September 2003): 283–93. doi:10.1016/s1471-0153(03)00024-2.

4) Weiss, Dara-Lynn. *The Heavy: A Mother, A Daughter, A Diet — a Memoir.* New York, New York: Ballantine Books, 2013.
5) Tylka, Tracy L., Julie C. Lumeng, and Ihuoma U. Eneli. "Maternal Intuitive Eating as a Moderator of the Association Between Concern about Child Weight and Restrictive Child Feeding." *Appetite,* 95 (December 2015): 158–65. doi:10.1016/j.appet.2015.06.023.
6) Cutting, Tanja M., Jennifer O. Fisher, Karen Grimm-Thomas, and Leann L. Birch. "Like Mother, Like Daughter: Familial Patterns of Overweight Are Mediated by Mothers' Dietary Disinhibition." *Journal of the American Academy of Child & Adolescent Psychiatry,* 38, no. 10 (October 1999): 1323. doi:10.1097/00004583-199910000-00028.
7) Blissett, J., E. Haycraft, and C. Farrow. "Inducing Preschool Children's Emotional Eating: Relations with Parental Feeding Practices." *American Journal of Clinical Nutrition,* 92, no. 2 (June 9, 2010): 359–65. doi:10.3945/ajcn.2010.29375.
8) Stephen, A, M Alles, C de Graaf, M Fleith, E Hadjilucas, E Isaacs, C Maffeis, et al. "The Role and Requirements of Digestible Dietary Carbohydrates in Infants and Toddlers." *European Journal of Clinical Nutrition,* 66, no. 7 (April 4, 2012): 765–79. doi:10.1038/ejcn.2012.27.
9) Kuzawa, C. W., H. T. Chugani, L. I. Grossman, L. Lipovich, O. Muzik, P. R. Hof, D. E. Wildman, et al. "Metabolic Costs and Evolutionary Implications of Human Brain Development." *Proceedings of the National Academy of Sciences* 111, no. 36 (August 25, 2014): 13010–15. doi:10.1073/pnas.1323099111.
10) De Graaf, Cees and Elizabeth H. Zandstra. "Sweetness Intensity and Pleasantness in Children, Adolescents,

and Adults." *Physiology & Behavior* 67, no. 4 (October 1999): 513–20. doi:10.1016/s0031-9384(99)00090-6.

11) Coldwell, Susan E., Teresa K. Oswald, and Danielle R. Reed. "A Marker of Growth Differs Between Adolescents with High Vs. Low Sugar Preference." *Physiology & Behavior*, 96, no. 4-5 (March 2009): 574–80. doi:10.1016/j.physbeh.2008.12.010.

12) Kroen, Gretchen Cuda. "Kids' Sugar Cravings Might Be Biological." September 26, 2011. Accessed October 9, 2016. http://www.npr.org/sections/thesalt/2011/09/26/140753048/kids-sugar-cravings-might-be-biological.

13) Jansen, Esther, Sandra Mulkens, Yvette Emond, and Anita Jansen. "From the Garden of Eden to the Land of Plenty. Restriction of Fruit and Sweets Intake Leads to Increased Fruit and Sweets Consumption in Children." *Appetite,* 51, no. 3 (November 2008): 570–75. doi:10.1016/j.appet.2008.04.012.

14) Kuijer, Roeline G., Jessica A. Boyce, and Emma M. Marshall. "Associating a Prototypical Forbidden Food Item with Guilt or Celebration: Relationships with Indicators of (un)healthy Eating and the Moderating Role of Stress and Depressive Symptoms." *Psychology & Health,* 30, no. 2 (September 29, 2014): 203–17. doi:10.1080/08870446.2014.960414.

15) Wadhera, Devina, Elizabeth D. Capaldi Phillips, Lynn M. Wilkie, and May M. Boggess. "Perceived Recollection of Frequent Exposure to Foods in Childhood Is Associated with Adulthood Liking." *Appetite,* 89 (June 2015): 22–32. doi:10.1016/j.appet.2015.01.011.

16) Satter, Ellyn. "Using Forbidden Food." 2016. Accessed October 13, 2016.

http://ellynsatterinstitute.org/htf/usingforbiddenfood. php.

17) Castle, Jill. "Fun Food & The 90:10 Rule." April 20, 2011. Accessed October 13, 2016. http://jillcastle.com/childhood-nutrition/fun-food-rules/.

Principle 4

1) Maimaran, Michal and Ayelet Fishbach. "If It's Useful and You Know It, Do You Eat? Preschoolers Refrain from Instrumental Food." *Journal of Consumer Research,* 41, no. 3 (October 1, 2014): 642–55. doi:10.1086/677224.

2) Zeinstra, Gertrude G, Maria A Koelen, Frans J Kok, and Cees de Graaf. "Cognitive Development and Children's Perceptions of Fruit and Vegetables; A Qualitative Study." *International Journal of Behavioral Nutrition and Physical Activity,* 4, no. 1 (2007): 30. doi:10.1186/1479-5868-4-30.

3) Tarabashkina, Liudmila, Pascale Quester, and Roberta Crouch. "Exploring the Moderating Effect of Children's Nutritional Knowledge on the Relationship Between Product Evaluations and Food Choice." *Social Science & Medicine,* 149 (January 2016): 145–52. doi:10.1016/j.socscimed.2015.11.046.

4) Frerichs, Leah, Loren Intolubbe-Chmil, Jeri Brittin, Kiersten Teitelbaum, Matthew Trowbridge, and Terry T. -K. Huang. "Children's Discourse of Liked, Healthy, and Unhealthy Foods." *Journal of the Academy of Nutrition and Dietetics,* 116, no. 8 (August 2016): 1323–31. doi:10.1016/j.jand.2016.01.014.

5) Finkelstein, Stacey R. and Ayelet Fishbach. "When Healthy Food Makes You Hungry." *Journal of*

Consumer Research, 37, no. 3 (October 2010): 357–67. doi:10.1086/652248.

6) Deci, Edward L., Richard Koestner, and Richard M. Ryan. "A Meta-Analytic Review of Experiments Examining the Effects of Extrinsic Rewards on Intrinsic Motivation." *Psychological Bulletin,* 125, no. 6 (1999): 627–68. doi:10.1037//0033-2909.125.6.627.

7) Goldsmith, Kelly, Eunice Kim Cho, and Ravi Dhar. "When Guilt Begets Pleasure: The Positive Effect of a Negative Emotion." *SSRN Electronic Journal, 49,* no. 6 (December 2012):872-881. doi:10.2139/ssrn.1917080.

8) Bellisle, F. and M. -F. Rolland-Cachera. "Three Consecutive (1993, 1995, 1997) Surveys of Food Intake, Nutritional Attitudes and Knowledge, and Lifestyle in 1000 French Children, Aged 9-11 Years." *Journal of Human Nutrition and Dietetics,* 13, no. 2 (April 2000): 101–11. doi:10.1046/j.1365-277x.2000.00222.x.

9) Lee, K., V. Talwar, A. McCarthy, I. Ross, A. Evans, and C. Arruda. "Can Classic Moral Stories Promote Honesty in Children?" *Psychological Science,* 25, no. 8 (June 13, 2014): 1630–36. doi:10.1177/0956797614536401.

10) Frerichs, Leah, Loren Intolubbe-Chmil, Jeri Brittin, Kiersten Teitelbaum, Matthew Trowbridge, and Terry T. K. Huang. "Children's Discourse of Liked, Healthy, and Unhealthy Foods." *Journal of the Academy of Nutrition and Dietetics,* 116, no. 8 (August 2016): 1323–31. doi:10.1016/j.jand.2016.01.014.

11) Gaier, Scott. "A Mindset for Learning: The Dispositions of Academically Successful Students." July 9, 2015. Accessed October 9, 2016. http://scholarlyteacher.com/2015/07/09/a-mindset-for-learning-the-dispositions-of-academically-successful-students/.

12) Borrelli, B, EM Tooley, and LA Scott-Sheldon. "Motivational Interviewing for Parent-Child Health

Interventions: A Systematic Review and Meta-Analysis." *Pediatric Dentistry,* 37, no. 3 (June 13, 2015): 254–65.

13) Peralta, Louisa R., Dean A. Dudley, and Wayne G. Cotton. "Teaching Healthy Eating to Elementary School Students: A Scoping Review of Nutrition Education Resources." *Journal of School Health,* 86, no. 5 (April 3, 2016): 334–45. doi:10.1111/josh.12382.

14) Dudley, Dean A, Wayne G Cotton, and Louisa R Peralta. "Teaching Approaches and Strategies That Promote Healthy Eating in Primary School Children: A Systematic Review and Meta-Analysis." *International Journal of Behavioral Nutrition and Physical Activity,* 12, no. 1 (February 25, 2015). doi:10.1186/s12966-015-0182-8.

15) Castle, Jill and Maryann Jacobsen. *Fearless Feeding: How to Raise Healthy Eaters from High Chair to High School.* San Francisco: Jossey-Bass, 2013.

16) Perikkou, Anastasia, Anna Gavrieli, Maria-Matina Kougioufa, Maria Tzirkali, and Mary Yannakoulia. "A Novel Approach for Increasing Fruit Consumption in Children." *Journal of the Academy of Nutrition and Dietetics,* 113, no. 9 (September 2013): 1188–93. doi:10.1016/j.jand.2013.05.024.

17) Fletcher, Margaret. *Discover Mindful Eating for Kids.* Shelly Skills 1st Edition, 2013.

Principle 5

1) Nicklaus, S. "The Role of Food Experiences During Early Childhood in Food Pleasure Learning." *Appetite,* 104 (August 25, 2015): 3–9. Accessed October 9, 2016. https://www.ncbi.nlm.nih.gov/pubmed/26298009.

2) Berge, J. M., S. Rowley, A. Trofholz, C. Hanson, M. Rueter, R. F. MacLehose, and D. Neumark-Sztainer. "Childhood Obesity and Interpersonal Dynamics During Family Meals." *Pediatrics,* 134, no. 5 (October 13, 2014): 923–32. doi:10.1542/peds.2014-1936.

3) Van der Horst, Klazine. "Overcoming Picky Eating. Eating Enjoyment as a Central Aspect of Children's Eating Behaviors." *Appetite,* 58, no. 2 (April 2012): 567–74. doi:10.1016/j.appet.2011.12.019.

4) L Hallberg, Bjorn-Rasmussen E, Rossander L, Suwanik R. "Iron Absorption from Southeast Asian Diets. II. Role of Various Factors that Might Explain Low Absorption." *Am J Clin Nutr,* 30, no. 4 (April 1977): 539-548.

5) Power, Michael L. and Jay Schulkin. "Anticipatory Physiological Regulation in Feeding Biology." *Appetite,* 50, no. 2-3 (October 24, 2007): 194-206.

6) Lewis, Mark. *The Biology of Desire.* New York, New York: Public Affairs, 2016.

7) Robert Batsell, W, Alan S Brown, Matthew E Ansfield, and Gayla Y Paschall. "'You Will Eat All of That!': A Retrospective Analysis of Forced Consumption Episodes." *Appetite,* 38, no. 3 (June 2002): 211–19. doi:10.1006/appe.2001.0482.

8) Cornil, Yann and Pierre Chandon. "Pleasure as an Ally of Healthy Eating? Contrasting Visceral and Epicurean Eating Pleasure and Their Association with Portion Size Preferences and Wellbeing." *Appetite,* 104 (September 2016): 52–59. doi:10.1016/j.appet.2015.08.045.

9) Vohs, K. D., Y. Wang, F. Gino, and M. I. Norton. "Rituals Enhance Consumption." *Psychological Science,* 24, no. 9 (July 17, 2013): 1714–21. doi:10.1177/0956797613478949.

10) Wood, Alex M., Jeffrey J. Froh, and Adam W. A. Geraghty. "Gratitude and Well-Being: A Review and Theoretical Integration." *Clinical Psychology Review,* 30, no. 7 (November 2010): 890–905. doi:10.1016/j.cpr.2010.03.005.

11) Froh, Jeffrey J., William J. Sefick, and Robert A. Emmons. "Counting Blessings in Early Adolescents: An Experimental Study of Gratitude and Subjective Well-Being." *Journal of School Psychology,* 46, no. 2 (April 2008): 213–33. doi:10.1016/j.jsp.2007.03.005.

12) Coulthard, Helen and Dipti Thakker. "Enjoyment of Tactile Play Is Associated with Lower Food Neophobia in Preschool Children." *Journal of the Academy of Nutrition and Dietetics,* 115, no. 7 (July 2015): 1134–40. doi:10.1016/j.jand.2015.02.020.

Principle 6

1) Golden, N. H., M. Schneider, and C. Wood. "Preventing Obesity and Eating Disorders in Adolescents." *Pediatrics,* 138, no. 3 (August 22, 2016): e20161649–e20161649. doi:10.1542/peds.2016-1649.

2) Neumark-Sztainer, Dianne, Melanie Wall, Mary Story, and Amber R. Standish. "Dieting and Unhealthy Weight Control Behaviors During Adolescence: Associations with 10-Year Changes in Body Mass Index." *Journal of Adolescent Health,* 50, no. 1 (January 2012): 80–86. doi:10.1016/j.jadohealth.2011.05.010.

3) Lowe, Michael R., Sapna D. Doshi, Shawn N. Katterman, and Emily H. Feig. "Dieting and Restrained Eating as Prospective Predictors of Weight Gain." *Frontiers in Psychology,* 4 (2013):517. doi:10.3389/fpsyg.2013.00577.

4) Sutin, A. R. and A. Terracciano. "Body Weight Misperception in Adolescence and Incident Obesity in Young Adulthood." *Psychological Science,* 26, no. 4 (March 5, 2015): 507–511. doi:10.1177/0956797614566319.

5) Robinson, E. and A. R. Sutin. "Parental Perception of Weight Status and Weight Gain Across Childhood." *Pediatrics,* 137, no. 5 (April 21, 2016): e20153957–e20153957. doi:10.1542/peds.2015-3957.

6) Eating Disorders Victoria. "Disordered Eating & Dieting." 2011. Accessed October 10, 2016. http://www.eatingdisorders.org.au/eating-disorders/disordered-eating-a-dieting.

7) Patton, G C, R Selzer, C Coffey, J B Carlin, and R Wolfe. "Onset of Adolescent Eating Disorders: Population Based Cohort Study over 3 Years." *BMJ,* 318, no. 7186 (March 20, 1999): 765–68. doi:10.1136/bmj.318.7186.765.

8) Ata, Rheanna N. and J. Kevin Thompson. "Weight Bias in the Media: A Review of Recent Research." *Obesity Facts,* 3, no. 1 (2010): 41–46. doi:10.1159/000276547.

9) Heuer, Chelsea. "Understanding the Complexity of Obesity." 2016. Accessed October 31, 2016. http://www.obesityaction.org/educational-resources/resource-articles-2/weight-bias/fattertainment-obesity-in-the-media.

10) Friedman, Roberta R and Rebecca M Puhl. "WEIGHT BIAS A Social Justice Issue A Policy Brief 2012." Yale Rudd Center for Food Policy and Obesity, 2012. http://www.uconnruddcenter.org/resources/upload/docs/what/reports/Rudd_Policy_Brief_Weight_Bias.pdf.

11) Puhl, R. M., J. L. Peterson, and J. Luedicke. "Weight-Based Victimization: Bullying Experiences of Weight Loss Treatment-Seeking Youth." *Pediatrics,* 131, no. 1

(December 24, 2012): e1–e9. doi:10.1542/peds.2012-1106

12) Udo, Tomoko and Carlos M. Grilo. "Perceived Weight Discrimination, Childhood Maltreatment, and Weight Gain in U.S. Adults with Overweight/Obesity. *Obesity*, 24, no. 6 (April 26, 2016): 1366–72. doi:10.1002/oby.21474.

13) Rachel Andrew, Marika Tiggemann, and Levina Clark. "Predictors of Intuitive Eating in Adolescent Girls." *Journal of Adolescent Health* 56, no. 2 (February 2015), doi:10.1016/j.jadohealth.2014.09.005.

14) Sutin, Angelina R. and Antonio Terracciano. "Perceived Weight Discrimination and Obesity." *PLoS ONE*, 8, no. 7 (July 24, 2013): e70048. doi:10.1371/journal.pone.0070048.

15) Murakami, Jessica M. and Janet D. Latner. "Weight Acceptance Versus Body Dissatisfaction: Effects on Stigma, Perceived Self-Esteem, and Perceived Psychopathology." *Eating Behaviors*, 19 (December 2015): 163–67. doi:10.1016/j.eatbeh.2015.09.010.

16) Andrew, Rachel, Marika Tiggemann, and Levina Clark. "Predictors and Health-Related Outcomes of Positive Body Image in Adolescent Girls: A Prospective Study." *Developmental Psychology*, 52, no. 3 (2016): 463–74. doi:10.1037/dev0000095.

17) Kater, Kathy. "The Model for Healthy Body Image and Weight." 2012. Accessed October 10, 2016. http://bodyimagehealth.org/model-for-healthy-body-image/.

18) Davis, Stan. "Advice for Youth." 2016. Accessed October 10, 2016. http://stopbullyingnow.com/advice-for-youth/.

19) Eli, Karin, Kyndal Howell, Philip A. Fisher, and Paulina Nowicka. "'Those Comments Last Forever': Parents and Grandparents of Preschoolers Recount How They

Became Aware of Their Own Body Weights as Children." *PLoS ONE,* 9, no. 11 (November 13, 2014): e111974. doi:10.1371/journal.pone.0111974.

20) Neff, Kristin. "Why We Should Stop Chasing Self-Esteem and Start Developing Self-Compassion." April 6, 2011. Accessed October 10, 2016. http://self-compassion.org/why-we-should-stop-chasing-self-esteem-and-start-developing-self-compassion/.

21) Sirois, Fuschia M., Ryan Kitner, and Jameson K. Hirsch. "Self-Compassion, Affect, and Health-Promoting Behaviors." *Health Psychology,* 34, no. 6 (2015): 661–69. doi:10.1037/hea0000158.

22) Zessin, Ulli, Oliver Dickhäuser, and Sven Garbade. "The Relationship Between Self-Compassion and Well-Being: A Meta-Analysis." *Applied Psychology: Health and Well-Being,* 7, no. 3 (August 26, 2015): 340–64. doi:10.1111/aphw.12051.

23) Homan, Kristin J. and Tracy L. Tylka. "Self-Compassion Moderates Body Comparison and Appearance Self-Worth's Inverse Relationships with Body Appreciation." *Body Image,* 15 (September 2015): 1–7. doi:10.1016/j.bodyim.2015.04.007.

Principle 7

1) Epstein, Robert. "What Makes a Good Parent? A Scientific Analysis Ranks the 10 Most Effective Child-Rearing Practices. Surprisingly, Some Don't Even Involve the Kids." November 1, 2010. Accessed October 12, 2016. http://www.scientificamerican.com/article.cfm?id=what-makes-a-good-parent.

2) Mischel, W, Y Shoda, and M. Rodriguez. "Delay of Gratification in Children." *Science,* 244, no. 4907 (May 26, 1989): 933–38. doi:10.1126/science.2658056.

3) Sominsky, Luba and Sarah J. Spencer. "Eating Behavior and Stress: A Pathway to Obesity." *Frontiers in Psychology,* 5 (May 13, 2014). doi:10.3389/fpsyg.2014.00434.

4) Francis, Lori A. and Elizabeth J. Susman. "Self-Regulation and Rapid Weight Gain in Children from Age 3 to 12 Years." *Archives of Pediatrics & Adolescent Medicine,* 163, no. 4 (April 6, 2009): 297. doi:10.1001/archpediatrics.2008.579.

5) Frankel, Leslie A., Sheryl O. Hughes, Teresia M. O'Connor, Thomas G. Power, Jennifer O. Fisher, and Nancy L. Hazen. "Parental Influences on Children's Self-Regulation of Energy Intake: Insights from Developmental Literature on Emotion Regulation." *Journal of Obesity,* 2012 (2012): 1–12. doi:10.1155/2012/327259.

6) American Psychologic Association. "Stress in America Press Room." 2016. Accessed November 1, 2016. http://www.apa.org/news/press/releases/stress/.

7) Anderson, S. E. and R. C. Whitaker. "Household Routines and Obesity in US Preschool-Aged Children." *Pediatrics,* 125, no. 3 (February 8, 2010): 420–28. doi:10.1542/peds.2009-0417.

8) Haines, Jess, Julia McDonald, Ashley O'Brien, Bettylou Sherry, Clement J. Bottino, Marie Evans Schmidt, and Elsie M. Taveras. "Healthy Habits, Happy Homes." *JAMA Pediatrics,* 167, no. 11 (November 1, 2013): 1072. doi:10.1001/jamapediatrics.2013.2356.

9) The Gottman Institute. "The Effectiveness of the Gottman Method - the Gottman Institute." 2016. Accessed October 12, 2016.

https://www.gottman.com/about/research/effectivene
ss-of-gottman-method/.
10) Mindful Staff. "Jon Kabat-Zinn: Defining
Mindfulness." January 11, 2016. Accessed October 12,
2016. http://www.mindful.org/jon-kabat-zinn-
defining-mindfulness/.
11) Zenner, Charlotte, Solveig Herrnleben-Kurz, and
Harald Walach. "Mindfulness-Based Interventions in
Schools-a Systematic Review and Meta-Analysis."
Frontiers in Psychology, 5 (June 30, 2014).
doi:10.3389/fpsyg.2014.00603.
12) Erickson, Jen. *MindUP™ Promotes Academic and
Social and Emotional Growth.* n.p., 2012.
http://www.interprofessional.ubc.ca/EarlyYears/docu
ments/A2_Pedrini_000.pdf.
13) O'Brien, Melli. "Six Ways to Teach Mindfulness to
Children - Mrs. Mindfulness." February 26, 2013.
Accessed October 12, 2016.
http://mrsmindfulness.com/how-to-teach-
mindfulness-to-children/.

Principle 8

1) Anderson, Sarah E. and Sarah A. Keim. "Parent–Child
Interaction, Self-Regulation, and Obesity Prevention in
Early Childhood." *Current Obesity Reports,* 5, no. 2
(April 1, 2016): 192–200. doi:10.1007/s13679-016-
0208-9.
2) Grobman, K. H. "Diana Baumrind & Parenting Styles."
2003. Accessed November 1, 2016.
http://www.devpsy.org/teaching/parent/baumrind_st
yles.html.
3) Newman, Kathy, Lynda Harrison, Carol Dashiff, and
Susan Davies. "Relationships Between Parenting Styles

and Risk Behaviors in Adolescent Health: An Integrative Literature Review." *Revista Latino-Americana de Enfermagem,* 16, no. 1 (February 2008): 142–50. doi:10.1590/s0104-11692008000100022.

4) Anderson, S. E., R. A. Gooze, S. Lemeshow, and R. C. Whitaker. "Quality of Early Maternal-Child Relationship and Risk of Adolescent Obesity." *Pediatrics,* 129, no. 1 (December 26, 2011): 132–40. doi:10.1542/peds.2011-0972.

5) Brown, Brene. "Shame V. Guilt - Brené Brown." January 14, 2013. Accessed November 1, 2016. http://brenebrown.com/2013/01/14/2013114shame-v-guilt-html/.

6) Lewis, Mark. *The Biology of Desire.* New York, New York: Public Affrairs, 2016.

7) Verstuyf, Joke, Heather Patrick, Maarten Vansteenkiste, and Pedro J Teixeira. "Motivational Dynamics of Eating Regulation: A Self-Determination Theory Perspective." *International Journal of Behavioral Nutrition and Physical Activity,* 9, no. 1 (2012): 21. doi:10.1186/1479-5868-9-21.

8) Berge, Jerica M., Melanie Wall, Nicole Larson, Katie A. Loth, and Dianne Neumark-Sztainer. "Family Functioning: Associations with Weight Status, Eating Behaviors, and Physical Activity in Adolescents." *Journal of Adolescent Health,* 52, no. 3 (March 2013): 351–57. doi:10.1016/j.jadohealth.2012.07.006.

9) TED. "What Makes a Good Life? Lessons from the Longest Study on Happiness | Robert Waldinger." *YouTube.* January 25, 2016. Posted October 12, 2016. https://www.youtube.com/watch?v=8KkKuTCFvzI.

10) Pace, Karen. "Wholehearted Parenting: Raising Kids with Courage and Resiliency." July 30, 2016. Accessed November 1, 2016.

http://msue.anr.msu.edu/news/wholehearted_parenti
ng_raising_kids_with_courage_and_resiliency.
11) Mind Tools Editorial Team. "Active Listening: Hear
What People Are Really Saying." Accessed October 12,
2016.
https://www.mindtools.com/CommSkll/ActiveListeni
ng.htm.
12) GoodTherapy. "'I' Message, 'I' Statement." August 4,
2014. Accessed October 12, 2016.
http://www.goodtherapy.org/blog/psychpedia/i-
message.
13) Milkie, Melissa A., Kei M. Nomaguchi, and Kathleen E.
Denny. "Does the Amount of Time Mothers Spend with
Children or Adolescents Matter?" *Journal of Marriage
and Family,* 77, no. 2 (March 4, 2015): 355–72.
doi:10.1111/jomf.12170.

Made in United States
North Haven, CT
14 May 2022

19182413R00117